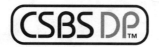

Infant-Toddler Checklist and Easy-Score™ User's Guide

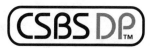

Infant-Toddler Checklist and Easy-Score™ User's Guide

Amy M. Wetherby, Ph.D., CCC-SLP
Florida State University
Tallahassee, Florida

and

Barry M. Prizant, Ph.D., CCC-SLP
Childhood Communication Services
Cranston, Rhode Island

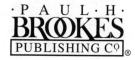

·P A U L ·H·
BR⊙⊙KES
PUBLISHING C⁰®

Baltimore • London • Sydney

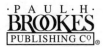

Paul H. Brookes Publishing Co.
Post Office Box 10624
Baltimore, Maryland 21285-0624
www.brookespublishing.com

Typeset by Auburn Associates, Baltimore, Maryland.
Manufactured in the United States of America by
Versa Press, Inc., East Peoria, Illinois.

Case studies and real names are used by permission.

The *CSBS DP™ Infant-Toddler Checklist and Easy-Score™ CD-ROM* and *User's Guide* are sold
together as ISBN 1-55766-560-5. A User's Guide without the CD-ROM can be purchased also
(ISBN 1-55766-655-5).

The following CSBS DP components can be purchased separately:
* *CSBS DP Manual, First Normed Edition*
* *CSBS DP Forms, First Normed Edition:* package includes 25 Infant-Toddler Checklists, 25
  Caregiver Questionnaires, 25 Behavior Sample: Scoring Worksheets, 25 Caregiver Perception
  Rating forms, 25 Infant-Toddler Checklist: Screening Reports, and 1 Outline of Sampling
  Procedures and Instructions card.
* *CSBS DP Caregiver Questionnaire:* package of 50

To order, contact Paul H. Brookes Publishing Co., Post Office Box 10624, Baltimore, Maryland
21285-0624 (1-800-638-3775; 410-337-9580; http://www.brookespublishing.com/csbsdp)
See pages 2–5 or the back of this manual for more information about the CSBS DP product
line. All products are available from Paul H. Brookes Publishing Co.

CD-ROM developed by TECHeGROUP, 535 Madison Avenue, Suite 404, Covington,
Kentucky 41011-1505. Technical questions may be addressed to support@TECHeGROUP.com
or by calling (800) 830-3387 9:00 A.M. to 5:00 P.M. eastern standard time. Your registration number is packaged with this book. You will need this number when you call for support. For more
information, see the Software License and Support Agreement on page 81.

Library of Congress Cataloging-in-Publication Data

Wetherby, Amy M.
    CSBS DP Infant-toddler checklist and Easy-Score user's guide / Amy M. Wetherby, Barry M.
Prizant.
        p. cm.
    Includes bibliographical references and index.
    ISBN 1-55766-560-5
    1. Communication and Symbolic Behavior Scales Developmental Profile. 2. Infants—
Psychological testing. 3. Toddlers—Psychological testing. I. Prizant, Barry, M. II. Title.

BF719.65.C65 W485 2003
155.42′236′0287—dc21

                                                                              2002038582

British Library Cataloging in Publication Data available from the British Library.

CONTENTS

ABOUT THE AUTHORS

Amy M. Wetherby, Ph.D., CCC-SLP, Laurel Schendel Professor of Communication Disorders, Department of Communication Disorders, Florida State University, Tallahassee, FL 32306

Dr. Wetherby received her doctorate from the University of California, San Francisco/Santa Barbara in 1982. She has more than 20 years of clinical experience in the design and implementation of communication programs for children with autism and severe communication impairments and is a Fellow of the American Speech-Language-Hearing Association. Dr. Wetherby's research has focused on communicative and cognitive-social aspects of language problems in children with autism and on the early identification of children with communication impairments. She has published extensively on these topics and presents regularly at national conventions. She is a co-author of the *Communication and Symbolic Behavior Scales* (with Barry M. Prizant; Paul H. Brookes Publishing Co., 1993) and *Communication and Symbolic Behavior Scales Developmental Profile* (with Barry M. Prizant; Paul H. Brookes Publishing Co., 2002) and co-editor of *Autism Spectrum Disorders: A Transactional Developmental Perspective* (with Barry M. Prizant; Paul H. Brookes Publishing Co., 2000).

Dr. Wetherby is the Project Director of the FIRST WORDS Project http://firstwords.fsu.edu) funded by a U.S. Department of Education Field-Initiated Research Grant on improving early identification of young children at risk for language and reading difficulties and a Model Demonstration Grant on early identification of communication disorders in infants and toddlers. She is also the Project Co-director (with Juliann Woods) of the Early Social Interaction Project funded by a U.S. Department of Education Model Demonstration Grant on the effectiveness of a comprehensive early intervention program for very young children with autism spectrum disorders. Dr. Wetherby served on the National Academy of Sciences Committee for Educational Interventions for Children with Autism and is the Executive Director of the Florida State University Center for Autism and Related Disabilities.

Barry M. Prizant, Ph.D., CCC-SLP, Adjunct Professor, Center for Human Development, Brown University, Providence, RI; Director, Childhood Communication Services, 2024 Broad Street, Cranston, RI 02905

Dr. Prizant has more than 25 years of experience as a clinical scholar, researcher, and consultant to young children with autism spectrum disorders (ASD) and other childhood disabilities and their families. He is Director of Childhood Communication Services, a private practice; an Adjunct Professor in the Center for Human Development at Brown University; and a Fellow of the American Speech-Language-Hearing Association. Formerly, he was an Associate Professor of Psychiatry in the Brown University Program in Medicine; Director of the Communication Disorders Department at Bradley Hospital in Providence, Rhode Island; and an Advanced Postdoctoral Fellow in Early Intervention at the University of North Carolina at Chapel Hill. He has developed and co-directed family-centered programs for newly diagnosed toddlers with ASD and their families in hospital and university clinic settings. Dr. Prizant is author or co-author of more than 90 articles and chapters, co-author of the *Communication and Symbolic Behavior Scales* (with Amy M. Wetherby; Paul H. Brookes Publishing Co., 1993) and *Communication and Symbolic Behavior Scales Developmental Profile* (with Amy M. Wetherby; Paul H. Brookes Publishing Co., 2002), co-editor of *Autism Spectrum Disorders: A Transactional Developmental Perspective* (with Amy M. Wetherby; Paul H. Brookes Publishing Co., 2000), and an editorial consultant for five professional journals in the areas of autism spectrum disorders and communication/language development and disorders. He has presented seminars and keynote addresses at conferences throughout North America, Europe, the Middle East, and the Far East. He also is an advisory board member of the Interdisciplinary Council on Developmental and Learning Disorders (Dr. Stanley Greenspan, Chair) and First Signs, Inc., an organization working to improve early diagnosis and referral. Dr. Prizant's current research and clinical interests include relationships between communication and social and emotional development, and identification and family-centered treatment of infants, toddlers, and young children who have or are at risk for social-communication difficulties, including ASD.

INTRODUCTION TO THE INFANT-TODDLER CHECKLIST AND EASY-SCORE

The Communication and Symbolic Behavior Scales Developmental Profile™ (CSBS DP™) Infant-Toddler Checklist is the first step in routine developmental screening for children ages 6–24 months. To help determine whether a developmental evaluation is needed, the Infant-Toddler Checklist asks families to answer 24 multiple-choice items, selecting from three to five choices for each item. The CSBS DP Infant-Toddler Checklist measures the following seven language predictors:

1. Emotion and eye gaze

2. Communication

3. Gestures

4. Sounds

5. Words

6. Understanding

7. Object use

The Checklist should be given to any family of a child between the ages of 6 and 24 months, regardless of whether that family has a concern about their child's development. The Checklist is to be completed by a caregiver, who may be either a parent or another person who nurtures the child on a daily basis. It takes about 5–10 minutes to complete. For caregivers who cannot answer the questions by reading them or writing the responses, the questions may be presented in an interview format with adequate explanations to clarify what is being asked. It is recommended that the Checklist be used to monitor development every 3 months between 6 and 24 months of age.

An accompanying CSBS DP Infant-Toddler Checklist: Family Information Form (see Appendix A) is used to collect family contact information for follow-up and information on birth and health history. The CSBS DP Infant-Toddler Checklist and CSBS DP Infant-Toddler Checklist: Family Information Form can be given to families in pediatricians' offices during well-child checkups or routine visits, in child care centers, or in other facilities serving infants and toddlers and their families.

The Checklist can be used independently or along with the other two components of the CSBS DP: 1) the four-page Caregiver Questionnaire for follow-up evaluation and 2) the 30-minute Behavior Sample for a face-to-face evaluation of the child (see Overview of CSBS DP, First Normed Edition). The Checklist is copyrighted (Paul H. Brookes Publishing Co., 2002) but remains free for use and can be printed from the Infant-Toddler Checklist and Easy-Score™ CD-ROM, downloaded from the Internet (www.bookespublishing.com/store/books/wetherbycsbsdp/checklist.htm) and freely photocopied, or duplicated by other methods.

The Checklist is to be completed by families or other caregivers but should be scored by health care or child care service providers. Because it is based on parent report, it is possible for the caregiver to overestimate or underestimate the child's abilities. Therefore, this tool should be used along with a brief observation of the child by a health care or child care service provider. Children who have scores in the concern range on any composite or the total score may have specific language impairments, hearing impairments, more general developmental delays, or autism spectrum disorder. With further development, they may only have speech impairments or they may catch up to children their age. The Checklist should only be used to decide that a developmental evaluation is needed.

The Infant-Toddler Checklist and Easy-Score software streamlines the scoring process and makes the Checklist a quick and efficient screening system. Simply input responses from the parent-completed Checklist, and the program calculates composite percentiles and standard scores based on embedded norms. The program automatically generates a screening report to add to the child's health record, and you can select from a menu of three letters to share personalized results and recommendations with the family. Caution should be taken not to alarm parents. We find that many parents already have concerns about their child, especially as their child is approaching age 18 months and is behind in language development. The early intervention literature emphasizes the notion of multiple risk factors; therefore, a child's scores on this Checklist need to be considered in relation to other known biological or environmental risk factors. Clinical judgment should be used in making decisions about the need for further evaluation with these scores as guidelines. Remember that the Checklist is not meant for a diagnostic evaluation and should not be used for a differential diagnosis.

OVERVIEW OF THE CSBS DP

The CSBS DP is a standardized tool designed to evaluate communication and symbolic abilities of children whose functional communication age is between 6 months and 2 years. It may also be used with preschool children whose chronological age is up to 5–6 years if their developmental level of functioning is younger than 24 months. The purpose of the CSBS DP is threefold:

1. For screening to identify children at risk for developmental delay or disability who need a developmental evauation

2. For evaluation to determine if a child has delays in social communication, expressive speech/language, and symbolic functioning

3. For evaluation to document changes in social communication, expressive speech/language, and symbolic functioning over time

Because of its brevity, the CSBS DP should not be used alone as the basis for decision making in program planning. It should be used as a guide to indicate areas that need further assessment or as an evaluation tool to monitor change. The Communication and Symbolic Behavior Scales™ (CSBS™), Normed Edition (Wetherby & Prizant, 1993), is a more in-depth tool and is designed for decision making in program planning.

Two-Step Screening and Evaluation Process

The CSBS DP consists of three components:

1. One-page CSBS DP Infant-Toddler Checklist for screening

2. Four-page CSBS DP Caregiver Questionnaire for follow-up evaluation

3. Thirty-minute CSBS DP Behavior Sample for a face-to-face evaluation of the child

The Infant-Toddler Checklist, Caregiver Questionnaire, and all forms required for scoring them, as well as for scoring the Behavior Sample, are included in the test kit.

The CSBS DP is a two-step process—the first step is screening with the CSBS DP Infant-Toddler Checklist, and, if needed, the second step is evaluating with the CSBS DP Caregiver Questionnaire and CSBS DP Behavior Sample, as diagrammed in Figure 1.1.

What Does the CSBS DP Measure?

The CSBS DP screens and evaluates a child's social communication, expressive speech/language, and symbolic abilities based on parent report and face-to-face evaluation. Each of the three components measures seven cluster areas that are organized into three composites.

- Social Composite: Emotion and Eye Gaze, Communication, and Gestures

- Speech Composite: Sounds and Words

- Symbolic Composite: Understanding and Object Use

How is the CSBS DP Administered?

The CSBS DP Infant-Toddler Checklist and the CSBS DP Caregiver Questionnaire provide important information about a child's abilities based

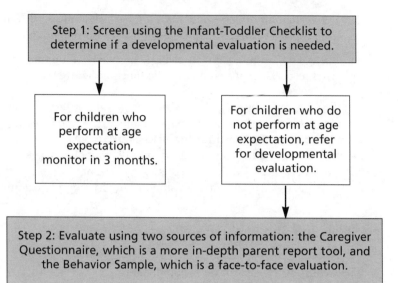

Figure 1.1. CSBS DP two-step process.

on caregiver report. The CSBS DP Behavior Sample is a face-to-face evaluation for professionals that uses a standard but flexible format for sampling behavior from young children. The sampling procedures consist of the following strategies designed to encourage spontaneous behavior. The strategies range in degree of structure provided by the adults.

- Communicative temptations, which are situations designed to entice a child to communicate
- Book sharing
- Symbolic play, using a feeding set to encourage pretending with objects
- Language comprehension probes
- Constructive play, using blocks to encourage stacking

Materials used during the CSBS DP Behavior Sample include action-based toys to entice spontaneous communication, books designed for young children, and play materials that evaluate how a child uses and plays with objects symbolically and constructively. Materials are presented in a designated sequence with minimal intrusion or direction. The child's behavior in order to encourage spontaneous communication and play. The caregiver is involved in the CSBS DP in three ways:

1. As a reporter and describer, by completing the CSBS DP Infant-Toddler Checklist and Caregiver Questionnaire

2. As a participant, by being present and interacting with the child during the CSBS DP Behavior Sample

3. As a validator, by completing the CSBS DP Behavior Sample: Caregiver Perception Rating to indicate how typical the child's behavior was during the sample

Who Can Administer the CSBS DP?

The CSBS DP can be administered by a certified speech-language pathologist, early interventionist, psychologist, or other professional trained to evaluate developmentally young children.

How Long Does it Take to Administer and Score?

The CSBS DP Infant-Toddler Checklist can be completed by a parent or caregiver in about 5–10 minutes. The CSBS DP Caregiver Questionnaire can be completed by a parent or caregiver in about 20 minutes and can be mailed ahead or given to the caregiver at the evaluation. The CSBS DP Behavior Sample takes about 30 minutes to complete, including a brief warm-up period in which both the child and caregiver should participate. The Behavior Sample can be scored during the sample by a trained evaluator. It may also be videotaped to document the child's performance and to enable the evaluator to score it later or to check the scoring. Video recording is not necessary unless the evaluator or parent wants to keep a recording, but it is recommended until the evaluator is experienced with the scoring procedures.

What Are the CSBS DP Materials?

The CSBS DP test kit includes:

- *CSBS DP Manual, First Normed Edition*

- Record forms for the CSBS DP Infant-Toddler Checklist, CSBS DP Caregiver Questionnaire, and CSBS DP Behavior Sample

- Carrying bag and materials for the Behavior Sample (these materials are a subset of those contained in the CSBS kit)

- Two tutorial videotapes for the Behavior Sample that contain six typically developing children; these tutorials demonstrate the sampling procedures and provide an opportunity for evaluators to practice scoring procedures.

WHY IS EARLY IDENTIFICATION IMPORTANT?

There is mounting evidence that intervention beginning during infancy or preschool has a greater impact on outcomes for children and families than providing services at school age (Barnett & Escobar, 1990). It is estimated that every dollar spent on early intervention can save $7.16 in later special education, crime, welfare, and other costs (Florida Starting Points, 1997). Despite federal mandates for early intervention, limitations in the identification process diminish children's access to services, and educators are not reaching most of the children and families who need help as early as they should (Meisels & Wasik, 1990). According to the *22nd Annual Report to Congress*, 11% of school-age children received special education services (U.S. Department of Education, 2000). In contrast, only 4.9% of preschool children received special education, and only 1.6% of infants and toddlers received early intervention services. These statistics indicate a significant need to improve early identification of children who are likely to require special education at school age.

Brain Research

Recent advances in brain research show how the environment sculpts the young child's brain, as neurons form connections and mature in response to stimulation. The environment has the greatest potential to influence a child's developing brain during the first few years of life. Early experiences affect brain structure because the brain operates on a "use it or lose it" principle (Carnegie Task Force on Meeting the Needs of Young Children, 1994; Ounce of Prevention Fund, 1996). If a child does not have adequate emotional, physical, cognitive, and language stimulation, neurons can be lost permanently.

School Readiness

Language development is one of the most critical school readiness skills. Children's capacity to talk and the size of their vocabulary when they enter kindergarten is predictive of success in school. Children with language problems in preschool are likely to face poor educational achievement at school age and are at increased risk to develop emotional and behavioral disorders (Baker & Cantwell, 1987; Prizant et al., 1990). Follow-up studies of preschoolers with speech and language problems consistently demonstrate persisting communication impairments in a substantial proportion of children and a high incidence of learning disabilities (Howlin & Rutter, 1987). Early intervention may prevent or decrease the severity of language delays in preschoolers, enhance school readiness, and increase later academic success in school.

Cumulative Effects of Poverty and Environmental Risk

Research on young children raised in poverty demonstrates the dramatic detrimental impact that impoverished environments can have on a child's capacity to learn to talk. Strong correlations exist among the amount of time that parents talk to their children, socioeconomic status, children's vocabulary, and children's IQ scores (Hart & Risley, 1992; Walker, Greenwood, Hart, & Carta, 1994). As documented by Hart and Risley, children's capacity for learning language is solidified by age 3, and the cumulative effects of the environment are evident. By school age, children in poverty are more likely to have developmental disabilities and behavior problems and to require special education services than other children (Brooks-Gunn & Duncan, 1997; U.S. Department of Education, 2000). Educational programs beginning at 3–4 years of age cannot hope to overcome such vast differences in cumulative experience. Educators are challenged to find ways to intervene even earlier in children's lives to effectively enhance child development and affect school readiness.

HOW CAN WE FIND CHILDREN EARLIER?

A child's level of communication development may be the best indicator of a developmental delay. Delays or disorders in communication development are the most prevalent symptom in children with disabilities (Wetherby & Prizant, 1996). When serious health or physical impairments are not present, a delay in language development may be the first evident symptom that a child is not developing typically. A language delay may be the primary problem or reflect delays in other domains (i.e., socioemotional, cognitive, motor, sensory).

There is a growing body of research indicating that prelinguistic abilities predict later language abilities. By their first birthday, children usually do not produce true words but can share attention and emotion and communicate intentionally using a variety of gestures and speech-like sounds that have shared meanings with caregivers (Bates, 1976; Bates, O 'Connell, & Shore, 1987; Stern, 1985). The readability of children's signals, coupled with contingent social responsiveness, facilitates successful acquisition of communication (Dunst, Lowe, & Bartholomew, 1990; Tronick, 1989). Typically, by their second birthday children use and understand hundreds of words, construct sentences, and engage in simple conversations. Linguistic communication begins when vocabulary growth accelerates, typically at about 19 months (Bates et al., 1987; Bloom, 1993). The dramatic changes in language abilities that occur from 1 to 2 years are reflected in the transition from prelinguistic to linguistic communication.

Although most children develop their first words between 12 and 15 months, it is common practice to wait until a child is at best 18–24 months, but usually at least 30 months of age, and still not talking to refer the child for an evaluation. The challenge for service providers determining whether to make a referral for a developmental evaluation is twofold. First, many children who are late in talking catch up on their own and need to be distinguished from children who will have persistent language problems. Second, children with delayed language skills need to be identified even earlier before language develops.

There is wide variation in the age and rate of acquisition of linguistic communication; however, this variation is strongly associated with prelinguistic development. A strong association has been found between children's prelinguistic gestures and sounds, communicative functions, comprehension of words, and use of objects in play at 1 year and language skills at 2 and 3 years (Paul, 1991; Paul & Jennings, 1992; Paul, Looney, & Dahm, 1991; Rescorla & Goosens, 1992; Thal & Tobias, 1992; Thal, Tobias, & Morrison, 1991; Wetherby et al., 1988). Many children are late in learning to talk, and many of these children do not need early intervention services. About 15% of 24-month-olds are late talkers with no other obvious delays (i.e., having fewer than 50 words or no word combinations; Rescorla, 1989, 1991). About half of these children show persisting problems in language development at age 3; the other half catch up with their peers spontaneously without intervention (Paul, 1991; Rescorla & Schwartz, 1990; Thal et al.,1991).

Research on preschoolers with language delays has important implications for distinguishing between children who will catch up spontaneously and those whose language problems are likely to persist. (For a review of this research, see McCathren, Warren, & Yoder, 1996; Olswang, Rodriguez, & Timler, 1998; and Wetherby & Prizant, 1992.) These studies have identified a collection of language predictors that are prelinguistic indicators of later language development and promise earlier and more accurate identification. The following seven language predictors have been identified:

1. Emotion and eye gaze

2. Rate and function of communication

3. Use of gestures

4. Use of sounds

5. Use of words

6. Understanding of words

7. Use of objects

These studies have demonstrated that children delayed only in the use of words are very likely to catch up on their own while children who are delayed also in several or many of the other predictors are likely to have persisting problems. Instead of waiting for children to start using words, evaluating these language predictors is a promising solution to improve early identification.

The literature reviewed previously suggests that a child's profile of communicative and symbolic abilities, even prior to the emergence of words, may be a sensitive indicator of the likelihood of subsequent difficulties in communication and language development. The findings for young children who show persisting language impairments indicate that measures of vocabulary alone are insufficient for early identification. Multiple measures across communicative and symbolic domains are necessary to identify and differentiate children who will outgrow their delay from those children who have specific versus more pervasive social or cognitive impairments. That is, a child who shows expressive language delays at 2 years and also shows delays in one or more of the other language predictors would be at a much higher risk than a child who demonstrates expressive language delays only.

These findings suggest greater urgency in initiating intervention that addresses delays, not only in expressive language, but also in other communicative and symbolic parameters. Because it is not yet possible to consider delays in expressive language for children younger than 18 months, it is even more critical to measure other parameters of communication and symbolic development in children younger than 18 months. Furthermore, patterns of strengths and weaknesses in the language predictors should provide critical information contributing to the early identification of a developmental disability. This empirical and theoretical framework forms the basis of the CSBS DP.

HOW CAN HEALTH CARE AND CHILD CARE PROVIDERS HELP?

Health care and child care providers can help in detecting communication problems earlier by giving the Infant-Toddler Checklist to parents of young children. We recommend that the Infant-Toddler Checklist be given to all families with children between 6 and 24 months of age every 3 months. However, some service providers may prefer only giving it to families who express concern about their child's development or who have children the service provider has concerns about. Caution should be used in giving the Checklist to families of children older than 24 months of age. For children older than 24 months, scores in the concern range would indicate the need for a developmental evaluation; however, scores that are not in the concern range would not necessarily indicate that the child is communicating as expected for his or her age.

When Should You Be Concerned If a Child Is Not Talking?

There is wide variation in the age that children begin talking and the rate that children learn to talk. This makes it difficult to decide when to be concerned if a child is not talking. The sounds and gestures children use to communicate and the ability to understand words and to play with objects provide important clues about the development of language. Following are some important milestones to help sort out which children to be concerned about:

- **9 months**: Children express pleasure by smiling and laughing while looking at an adult. They use gestures and sounds to get help or attention.

- **12 months:** Children respond by looking when an adult calls their name. At this age they use a variety of sounds and gestures to communicate and begin to use a few words. They are interested in doing things with objects, such as trying to drink out of a cup, eat with a spoon, or brush with a hairbrush.

- **15 months**: Children are using lots of sounds, gestures, and a few words to communicate. Many will ask for help, show off, and point out interesting things to adults. They can follow simple directions and can stack two to three blocks.

- **18 months:** Words are becoming the primary way many children at this age communicate. They can make more than five different consonant sounds (like m, n, p, b, t, and d) and are using more than 10 different words. They are beginning to pretend with objects (e.g., pretending to feed a doll or stuffed animal).

- **24 months**: Children usually use more than 50 words and combine words together to make simple sentences. They can put several actions together in their play, such as stirring, scooping, and feeding a doll with a spoon.

What If Families Have Concerns?

Families are often the first to raise concerns about their child's development. Concerns raised by the majority of families are warranted, and therefore, it is important to give the Infant-Toddler Checklist to any family that has any concern about their child's communication development. Some families have concerns about their child, but their child is developing typically. It is important to reassure those families and answer questions that they may have about their child's development. For these families, their child's development can be monitored with the Infant-Toddler Checklist or other components of the CSBS DP to make sure their child is progressing as expected and to provide information about typical development.

What If Families Are Not Yet Concerned?

Some children have delays but families are not yet concerned. It can be difficult for parents to learn that their child is not developing as expected. It is important not to alarm families and to offer support as concerns are raised. It can be confusing to families if one professional tells them that their child is doing fine and another indicates concern. Health care providers can help by becoming familiar with early indicators of communication problems and establishing collaborative relationships with professionals who are experienced with developmental evaluations of young children for referrals. If intervention can be provided early, the child's chances for improvement are much greater.

EASY-SCORE ADMINISTRATION PROCEDURES

This chapter walks you through the Easy-Score program, giving step-by-step instructions.

TO INSTALL THE EASY-SCORE PROGRAM

Place the CD-ROM into the disk drive. Wait. The CD will start automatically. Follow the steps on the screen (see Figure 2.1). A copy of the licensing agreement also appears in this manual in Appendix E for your reference. If the setup does not automatically initiate, then double click on the My Computer icon on your desktop. Next, double click on the icon for your CD-ROM drive (this can be any letter from D though Z). Then, double-click on "setup.exe," and the program will begin the installation process.

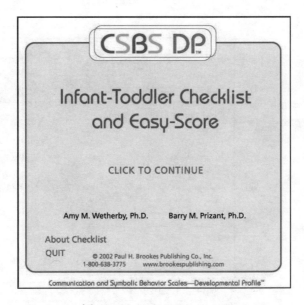

Figure 2.1.   Opening screen of the Easy-Score program.

TO ENTER A NEW CHECKLIST RECORD

Step 1: Entering Child Information

Go to the Menu page and select the "Enter a new Checklist record" button. This will take you to the Child Information page (see Figure 2.2). Fill in each field, pressing tab after you enter the information to move to the next field. If you make any errors while entering the information, then you can use the mouse to select the field with the error and reenter the data. For "Examiner's name," enter the physician or other professional who will be discussing the recommendations with the child's caregivers. Remember, the names as entered on the Child Information page will appear in the letter to be sent to the caregivers.

When you reach "Was child's birth premature?", you will need to click to select the correct response—yes or no—using your mouse. Select "Yes" if the child was more than 4 weeks premature. If the answer is "No," then you will proceed to the next page to enter the Checklist responses (see Step 2).

If the answer is "Yes," you must then respond to the question "How many weeks premature?" by clicking on the gray box and typing in the number of weeks. The "Chronological age in months" will display the corrected age when you press the tab key on your keyboard. The age will also be corrected if you proceed to the next page immediately after entering the number of weeks the child's birth was premature. If a child's birth was premature, then the reports, letters, and database file will all indicate "This is a corrected age."

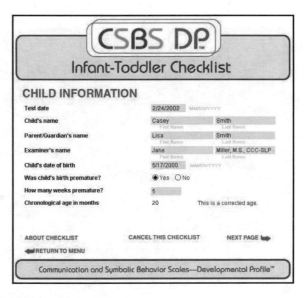

Figure 2.2.   Child information page.

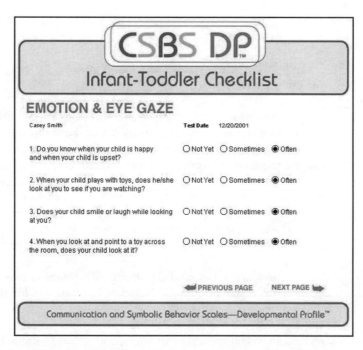

Figure 2.3.   Filling out the checklist.

The links at the bottom of the screen help you navigate through the program as follows:

- The "About Checklist" button provides contact information for reordering or support.

- The "Cancel This Checklist" button resets the screen to a blank Child Information page, and any information entered will be lost.

- The "Next Page" button will move you forward through the Checklist.

- The "Return to Menu" button takes you to the main menu pages, and any information entered will be lost.

Step 2: Entering Checklist Responses

Once you have the Child Information input, it is time to transfer the caregiver's responses from the Infant-Toddler Checklist to the electronic database by using your mouse to click on the circle indicating the correct response on screen. The on-screen Checklist has been divided into the clusters for easier data entry:

- Emotion and Eye Gaze (see Figure 2.3)

- Communication

- Gestures

- Sounds
- Words
- Understanding
- Object Use

You can use the "Next Page" and "Previous Page" buttons at the bottom of your screen to move forward and backward through the Checklist. **However, the "Next Page" option will not appear until all questions on the page have been answered.** When you have completed entering the responses to all of the questions, the Easy-Score program will automatically generate a Screening Report (see Figure 2.4).

On the Screening Report, a raw score will be tallied for each of the seven clusters, the Social, Speech, and Symbolic Composites, as well as for the Total Score. The total possible points for the raw scores are listed in Table 2.1.

A Standard Score and the Percentile Rank will be tallied for the Social, Speech, and Symbolic Composites as well as for the Total Score. The standard scores for the three Composites are based on a mean of 10 and a standard deviation of 3. The standard scores for the Total is based on a mean of 100 and a standard deviation of 15. The relationship between the standard scores for the Composites and Total and percentile ranks are shown in Table 2.2.

If the child's Standard Score in any of these areas falls 1.25 standard deviations below the mean and the child's Percentile Rank is at or below 10, then a red "Yes" appears in the Concern column.

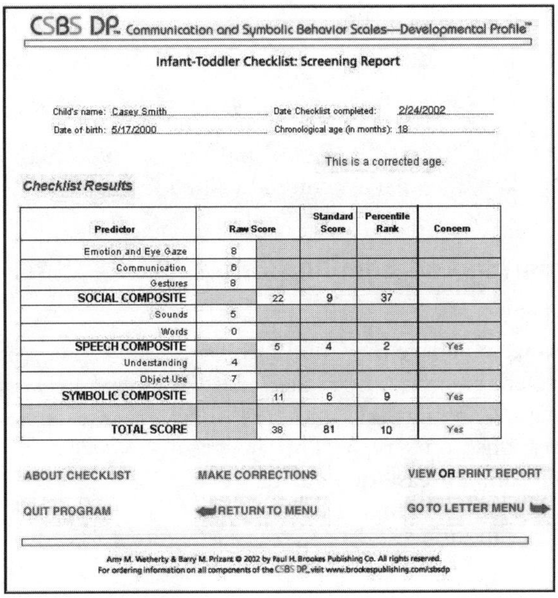

CSBS DP. Communication and Symbolic Behavior Scales—Developmental Profile™

Infant-Toddler Checklist: Screening Report

Child's name: _Casey Smith_   Date Checklist completed: _2/24/2002_
Date of birth: _5/17/2000_   Chronological age (in months): _18_

This is a corrected age.

Checklist Results

Predictor	Raw Score	Standard Score	Percentile Rank	Concern
Emotion and Eye Gaze	8			
Communication	8			
Gestures	9			
SOCIAL COMPOSITE		22	9	37
Sounds	5			
Words	0			
SPEECH COMPOSITE		5	4	2	Yes
Understanding	4			
Object Use	7			
SYMBOLIC COMPOSITE		11	6	9	Yes
TOTAL SCORE		38	81	10	Yes

ABOUT CHECKLIST   MAKE CORRECTIONS   VIEW OR PRINT REPORT

QUIT PROGRAM   ◄ RETURN TO MENU   GO TO LETTER MENU ►

Ann M. Wetherby & Barry M. Prizant © 2002 by Paul H. Brookes Publishing Co. All rights reserved.
For ordering information on all components of the CSBS DP, visit www.brookespublishing.com/csbsdp

Figure 2.4.   Screening Report generated by the Easy-Score program.

Table 2.1. Total possible points for each Cluster, Composite, and Total on the Infant-Toddler Checklist.

Composite	Possible Points
SOCIAL COMPOSITE:	
Emotion and Eye Gaze	8
Communication	8
Gestures	10
	26
SPEECH COMPOSITE:	
Sounds	8
Words	6
	14
SYMBOLIC COMPOSITE:	
Understanding	6
Object Use	11
	17
SOCIAL COMPOSITE:	26
SPEECH COMPOSITE:	14
SYMBOLIC COMPOSITE:	17
TOTAL	57

Table 2.2. Standard deviations (SD), standard scores (SS), and percentile ranks (PR) for the Composites and Total scores

SD	Composite SS	Total SS	PR
	17	135	99
+2 SD	16	130	98
	15	125	95
	14	120	91
+1 SD	13	115	84
	12	110	75
	11	105	63
MEAN	10	100	50
	9	95	37
	8	90	25
−1 SD	7	85	16
	6	80	9
	5	75	5
−2 SD	4	70	2
	3	65	1

The links at the bottom of the Screening Report help you navigate through the program as follows:

- The "About Checklist" button provides contact information for reordering or support.

- The "Make Corrections" button takes you to the Edit Child Information page containing the data originally entered (see Figure 2.5). Click to select the field with the error, and enter the corrected information. If the child's chronological age in months is affected due to the correction, then the program will modify the screening report to reflect the revised Standard Scores, Percentile Rank, and Concern rating for the corrected age. If the child's chronological age is incorrect due to an error in the test date entered, the child's date of birth entered, or the response to "Was the child's birth premature?", then reenter the data. Once entered, the corrected information will be reflected on the screening reports, in the parent letters, and in the database record for the child. From the Edit Child Information page, you can return to the menu and the corrections will be saved, you can page through the Checklist to ensure the data entered corresponds to the caregiver's responses, or you can go directly to the report page to review the revised screening report.

- The "View or Print Report" button lets you view the complete Screening Report, including the Referral Recommendation and an explanation of criteria levels, or print the complete Screening Report. When you are viewing the complete Screening Report, you can use your mouse to scroll down to review the recommendations. You have the options to print out the report for your records, make corrections, or return to Menu. Selecting the "Print Report" option will bring up the print command box allowing you to specify the number of copies to be printed and will ask you whether you want to print the Current Record, Blank Record, showing fields, and Records Being Browsed.

- The "Quit Program" or "Return to Menu" buttons allow you to exit this screen while saving the child's record in the database.

- The "Go to the Letter Menu" button shows you the three letters that can be generated to inform caregivers of your referral recommendation of the screening results.

   If an error is discovered when reviewing the Checklist responses, click on the appropriate circle to alter the response. All responses entered into the electronic database must correspond to the answers provided by the caregivers. Clinicians may use their professional judgment in determining the referral recommendation when sharing results with the caregivers, but the database should reflect the caregivers' perceptions of their children's development.

Step 3: Finalizing the Screening
Report and Generating a Parent Letter

After you are sure all errors are corrected and have printed a copy of the child's Screening Report, the software takes you to the Parent Letter

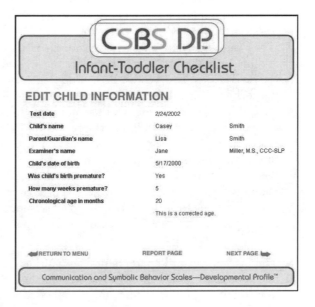

Figure 2.5.   Editing child information page.

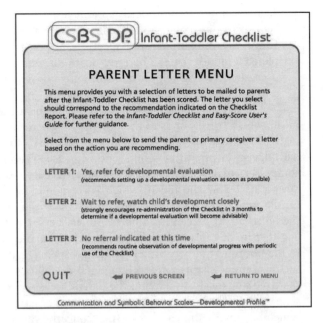

Figure 2.6.   Parent letter menu page.

Menu screen (see Figure 2.6). The Parent Letter Menu provides you with a selection of letters that summarize the recommendation based on the Infant-Toddler Checklist results. The letter to parents does not include scores but briefly explains what the Checklist measures, whether a developmental evaluation is recommended, and, if so, why this evaluation is important. A letter should be sent to every parent within 1 week of completion of the Infant-Toddler Checklist.

We have developed three different versions of the letter to parents that the user can select based on the recommendation made. The first letter is for children who perform in the "no concern" range on all three composites and indicates that the child is currently communicating as expected for his or her age and that the child should be monitored with another Checklist in 3 months (see Figure 2.7). The second letter is for children who perform in the "concern" range on the Speech Composite only for the first time and recommends that the child should be monitored with another Checklist in 3 months (see Figure 2.8). The third letter is for children who perform in the "concern" range on the Social and/or Symbolic Composite or for children who have performed in the "concern" range on the Speech Composite for the second time and recommends referring the child for a developmental evaluation (see Figure 2.9).

The letter you select should correspond to the pattern of scores indicated on the Screening Report. Based on our validation studies summarized in Chapter 7 of the CSBS DP Manual and Chapter 3 of this manual, we have determined that the following recommendation should be made, depending on the child's pattern of scores:

• A child should be referred for an evaluation if the Social Composite, Symbolic Composite, or the Total Score are in the concern range.

- A child should be monitored carefully if the Speech Composite is in the "concern" range and should be referred for an evaluation if the Speech Composite remains in the "concern" range on a second Checklist completed 3 months later. The Easy-Score Program is designed so that the user can decide which of the three letters to send to the parent.

The cutoff for concern was set at 1.25 standard deviations below the mean, which corresponds to the bottom 10th percentile, based on our validation studies. (See Table 2.2 to understand the relationship between standard deviations, standard scores, and percentile ranks.) We recognize that some users may prefer a more conservative cutoff score of 1.5 standard deviations below the mean, which corresponds to the bottom 7th percentile, or 2.0 standard deviations below the mean, which corresponds to the bottom 2nd percentile, whereas other users may prefer a more liberal cutoff score of 1.0 standard deviations below the mean, which corresponds to the bottom 16th percentile. Many factors may enter into this decision, such as family history of developmental disabilities, environmental risks, the child's medical history, and the parent's level of concern as well as the state criteria for eligibility for early intervention services. It is important to remember that if the child is in the "concern" range on only the Speech Composite, it is necessary to examine the previous Infant-Toddler Checklist scores, if available, to determine which letter to give.

At this point, you have the option of printing one of three letters, returning to the previous screen (Screening Report page), or quitting the program. When you choose any of the options offered, the child's data will automatically be saved in the database.

Re: (CSBS DP) Infant-Toddler Checklist

Child's name: Casey Smith
Date of birth: 5/17/2000
Date Checklist completed: 02/24/2002
Chronological age (in months): 20
Referral recommended: Not Yet

Dear Lisa Smith:

Thank you for taking the time to complete the Infant-Toddler Checklist. The Checklist was used to screen your child's ability to communicate using eye gaze, gestures, sounds, or words and to play with toys.

Based on the information you provided on the Checklist, your child is currently communicating as expected for his or her age. Because new skills are emerging each month, it is important to monitor Casey's development, and we would like you to complete the Checklist again in about 3 months. We will contact you at the appropriate time to provide you with a Checklist. If you have any questions or concerns about your child's development, please feel free to call us. We look forward to assisting you.

Sincerely,

Jane Miller, M.S., CCC-SLP

Figure 2.7.   Letter to parents with referral not recommended.

Re: (CSBSDP) Infant-Toddler Checklist

Child's name: Casey Smith
Date of birth: 5/17/2000
Date Checklist completed: 02/24/2002
Chronological age (in months): 20
Referral recommended: Not Yet

Dear Lisa Smith:

Thank you for taking the time to complete the Infant-Toddler
Checklist. The Checklist was used to screen your child's ability to
communicate using eye gaze, gestures, sounds, or words and to
play with toys.

Based on the information you provided on the Checklist, we are
recommending that your child's development be monitored so we
can see how Casey's skills are emerging. We would like you to
complete the Checklist again in about 3 months. We will contact
you at the appropriate time to provide you with a Checklist. If you
have any questions or concerns about your child's development,
please feel free to call us. We look forward to assisting you.

Sincerely,

Jane Miller, M.S., CCC-SLP

Figure 2.8.   Letter to parents with referral not yet recommended, but need for ongoing monitoring.

Re: (CSBSDP) Infant-Toddler Checklist

Child's name: Casey Smith
Date of birth: 5/17/2000
Date Checklist completed: 02/24/2002
Chronological age (in months): 20
Referral recommended: Yes

Dear Lisa Smith:

Thank you for taking the time to complete the Infant-Toddler Checklist. The
Checklist was used to screen (child's name)'s ability to communicate using
eye gaze, gestures, sounds, or words and to play with toys.

Based on the information you provided on the Checklist, we are recommending that Casey be referred for a developmental evaluation. Please call our
office so we can help make these arrangements.

The Checklist does not conclusively determine if your child has a
problem in development, but indicates whether further evaluation or follow-
up is needed. A more thorough developmental evaluation can determine if
Casey has a communication delay. If needed, we will provide information for
planning the next steps to support you and your child. Children who have
early communication delays may have difficulties in other areas of development. It is important to catch communication problems in young children as
early as possible, as early intervention services may remediate or lessen the
impact of communication problems and help you support your child's development. We look forward to assisting you.

Sincerely,

Jane Miller, M.S., CCC-SLP

Figure 2.9.   Letter to parents with referral recommended.

TO FIND PREVIOUS CHECKLIST RECORDS

Once entered, a child's information and Checklist is stored in the Easy-
Score database. To access a specific database file, select "Find Previous

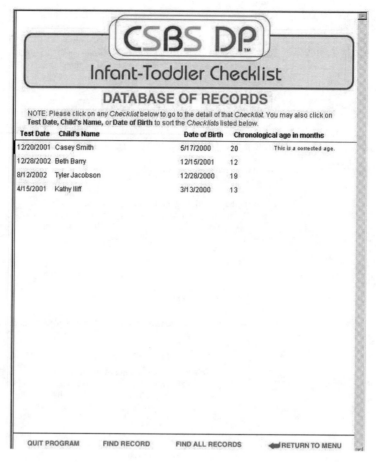

Figure 2.10. Database of records.

Checklist Records." The Child Information page will pop up to streamline your search for existing records. You have the option to search for a child's record by the date the test was administered, by the child's name, by the child's date of birth, or by the child's chronological age in months:

- Searching by the child's name is the easiest way to directly access a specific child's record.

- Searching by the test date will pull up every child's record whose test was completed on that date.

- Searching by a child's date of birth or chronological age in months will display records for all children whose test was administered at that age or born on that day.

Enter information in any of the available fields and then click the "Continue Find" button at the bottom right hand corner of the screen to review a list of records meeting your search criteria. Do not hit Return or Enter at this point. You must use the "Continue Find" button to proceed.

You can bypass the search page [Child Information page] by clicking "Go To Database" to see a full listing of the Checklists that have been entered. You may also click on any of the headings—Test Date, Child's Name, or Child's Date of Birth—to sort the Checklist listings displayed. You can also clear the data you've entered in the search fields and open a blank Child Information page by clicking on "New Search."

Once the corresponding records have been pulled (see Figure 2.10), click on the desired listing to view the child's Infant-Toddler Checklist: Screening Report page. Other options on the Database of Records screen include

- "Quit Program" to close the Easy-Score software

- "Find Record" to return to the Child Information page to refine your search criteria

- "Find All Records" to access a full listing of all Checklist records entered in the database

- "Return to Menu" to take you back to the main menu page

TECHNICAL CHARACTERISTICS ⟨ 3 ⟩

This chapter describes the technical characteristics of the CSBS DP Infant-Toddler Checklist. The first part of this chapter addresses the characteristics of the sample used for standardization. The remainder of the chapter examines data on the reliability and validity of the CSBS DP.

For a full discussion of the development and technical characteristics of the CSBS DP, see the *Communication and Symbolic Behavior Scales Developmental Profile (CSBS DP) Manual, First Normed Edition* (Wetherby & Prizant, 2002).

STANDARDIZATION

The First Normed Edition of the CSBS DP was standardized from 1997 to 2000. The standardization consisted of collecting Infant-Toddler Checklists for children and scoring each to derive norms. A parent or other caregiver knowledgeable about the child completed the CSBS DP Infant-Toddler Checklists.

Standardization Sample

A total of 2,188 Infant-Toddler Checklists were included in the standardization sample. Children were recruited for the standardization sample from a total of eight sites in the United States and two sites in Canada; however, the majority of children in the standardization sample were recruited from the Tallahassee, Florida, region. Therefore, although the standardization sample is large, it is not a nationally representative sample. Sources for recruiting children included doctor's offices, child care centers, and health fairs or other community events and sites regularly attended by families of young children. Children with known developmental delays or who qualified for Part C early intervention services were excluded from the standardization sample but were included in some validation studies. Because of the extent of the under-identification of children with developmental delays from birth to 24 months of age, it is presumed that at least 10% of the standardization sample has developmental delays or disabilities, although children with severe disabilities are likely not included in this sample.

The children ranged in age from 6 to 24 months for the CSBS DP Infant-Toddler Checklist sample. Because it was expected that the CSBS DP would be used more than once in screening and evaluating children's communication and symbolic behavior over the course of several months, approximately 15% of the standardization sample was retested within an average of 2–3 months after the initial administration. These second administrations were included in the normative scores because, as Angoff (1971) pointed out, they increase the relevance of the norms to their intended use and reduce the error that would be associated with estimates of developmental improvement based on different children at different ages. This method of data collection made it possible to create data sets that include both cross-sectional and longitudinal data. (For more detail on the retested children, see the discussion of stability later in this chapter.)

The standardization sample is described in Tables 3.1–3.6 for several important demographic variables, including child's age at CSBS DP administration (Table 3.1), gender (Table 3.2), race (Table 3.3), Hispanic origin (Table 3.4), and parent age and education (Tables 3.5 and 3.6).

Age

Table 3.1 shows the number of children and the percentage of the total standardization sample at each age interval for the CSBS DP Infant-Toddler Checklist. The children are grouped according to age in intervals that correspond with the norms presented in Appendix C. For the Infant-

Table 3.1. Children in the standardization sample, by age in months

Age (months)	n	Percent of total
6	50	2.3
7	42	1.9
8	77	3.5
9	126	5.8
10	86	3.9
11	312	14.3
12	296	13.5
13	121	5.5
14	128	5.9
15	174	8.0
16	98	4.5
17	99	4.5
18	133	6.1
19	107	4.9
20	84	3.8
21	87	4.0
22	82	3.7
23	50	2.3
24	36	1.6
Total	2188	100.0

Table 3.2. Children in the standardization sample, by gender

Gender	n	Percent of total
Female	1090	49.8
Male	1098	50.2
Total	**2188**	**100.0**

Toddler Checklist, norms are presented in 1-month intervals from 6 to 24 months of age. As can be seen, most of the age intervals include at least 60 children and many include more than 100 children.

Gender

Table 3.2 shows the number of children by gender for the Infant-Toddler Checklist. This table shows an almost equal balance of males and females for the CSBS DP Infant-Toddler Checklist.

Race and Ethnicity

Tables 3.3 and 3.4 show the number and percentage of children in the standardization sample by race and Hispanic origin for the Infant-Toddler Checklist. The majority of children in the standardization sample were Caucasian; however, a substantial number of African American children were included in the standardization sample for the Infant-Toddler Checklist, well above the percentage in the U.S. population, based on 2000 population estimates from the U.S. Census Bureau. The reason that the percentage of African American children is so high for the Infant-Toddler Checklist is that a large proportion of the sample was drawn from the Tallahassee region, and approximately one fourth of the population in that region is African American. Thus, African American children are over-represented in the standardization samples for the Infant-Toddler Checklist. The proportion of children in the standardization sample who were of Hispanic origin is below that represented on average in the United States, based on the 2000 Census data. The proportions reported in Tables 3.3 and 3.4 indicate that the standardization sample has adequate racial diversity but that individuals of Hispanic origin are under-represented.

Table 3.3. Children in the standardization sample, by race

Race	U.S. population[a] Percent of total		Infant-Toddler Checklist n	Percent of total
White	75.1		1504	71.5
Black	12.3		483	23.0
Asian	3.6		61	2.9
Other	8.9		56	2.7
Total	**100.0**		**2104**	**100.0**

[a]Based on 2000 U.S. Bureau figures

Table 3.4. Children in the standardization sample, by Hispanic origin

	U.S. population[a] Percent of total	Infant-Toddler Checklist	
Hispanic		*n*	Percent of total
Yes	12.5	120	5.5
No	87.5	2068	94.5
Total	**100.0**	**2188**	**100.0**

[a]Based on 2000 U.S. Census Bureau figures

Parent Age and Education

Table 3.5 shows the average age and amount of education for parents of children in the standardization sample for the Infant-Toddler Checklist because these variables are strongly indicative of socioeconomic class. Table 3.5 reports the average ages of the mother and father at the time of the child's birth in years. It also reports the average number of years of education for the mother and father, ranging from 8, indicating completion of eighth grade, to 22, indicating completion of twelfth grade plus 4 years of undergraduate school and 6 years of graduate or medical school.

Table 3.6 shows the amount of education for the mothers and fathers of children in the standardization sample for the Infant-Toddler Checklist in relation to the 2000 U.S. Census Bureau figures, based on completion of less than high school, high school, some college, and a college degree. The proportions reported in Table 3.6 indicate that the education level of the parents of children in the standardization sample is above the national average.

The demographic information reported in Tables 3.5 and 3.6 suggests that the socioeconomic level of these families is above the national average. *Therefore, caution should be taken when using the norms for the CSBS DP with parents who have low education levels, particularly those who have not completed high school.*

Table 3.5. Parent's age at childbirth and years of education for children in standardization sample

	Infant-Toddler Checklist
Mother's age	
Mean	29.3
Standard deviation	6.0
Range	12.6–45.5
Father's age	
Mean	31.7
Standard deviation	7.1
Range	14.3–60.9
Mother's education	
Mean	14.7
Standard deviation	2.2
Range	8–21
Father's education	
Mean	14.6
Standard deviation	2.6
Range	8–22

Table 3.6. Children of the standardization sample, by parent's education

	U.S. population[a] Percent of total	Infant-Toddler Checklist n	Percent of total
Mother's education			
Some high school or less	15.0	79	3.8
High school diploma	29.2	444	21.4
Some college	34.4	473	22.8
College degree	21.5	1082	52.1
Total	**100.0**	**2078**	**100.0**
Father's education			
Some high school or less	18.4	82	4.2
High school diploma	31.8	553	28.0
Some college	30.6	373	18.9
College degree	19.2	965	48.9
Total	**100.0**	**1973**	**100.0**

[a]Based on 2000 U.S. Census Bureau figures for 18- to 34-year-olds

DEVELOPMENT OF NORMATIVE SCORES

The development of norms required a balance of concern for several elements of CSBS DP construction, including the wide variety of communication and symbolic behavior parameters rated, the uneven growth of these parameters within the age range of the standardization sample, the variability with the obtained sample, and the intended use of the CSBS DP norms in comparing observed and expected performance not only for children within but also outside the age range of the standardization group.

The first step was to generate scores that would aid in interpretation of various patterns of performance on related items. These scores, called cluster scores, are based on summing the raw scores for meaningful combinations of items. The CSBS DP Infant-Toddler Checklist has seven clusters for each of the components that correspond to the other components of the CSBS DP.

1. Emotion and Eye Gaze
2. Communication
3. Gestures
4. Sounds
5. Words
6. Understanding
7. Object Use

The cluster scores were calculated using the raw scores for the 24 items of the CSBS DP Infant-Toddler Checklist. Because the Infant-Toddler Checklist has a small number of items and range of scores within each cluster, norms were not created at the level of the cluster scores for the Infant-Toddler Checklist. The scores for the seven clusters were summed to create three composites, named for simplicity as Social, Speech, and Symbolic, and a total. The composites were derived from the clusters as follows:

- Social (sum of Emotion and Eye Gaze, Communication, and Gestures)
- Speech (sum of Sounds and Words)
- Symbolic (sum of Understanding and Object Use)

The resulting sum for each combination of items was then obtained for each child in the standardization sample, and a frequency distribution for each of the combined raw scores was obtained for each age interval. Percentile ranks derived from each frequency distribution were then converted, using a table of the normal curve, to normalized standard scores with a mean of 10 and a standard deviation of 3 for each composite and a mean of 100 and a standard deviation of 15 for the total. Some smoothing was performed to adjust for sampling irregularities on all intervals studied; however, the age intervals for most combined scores exhibited adequately stable increases over the age range so that they were chosen for use.

The percentile ranks and standard scores for each of the three components of the Infant-Toddler Checklist are presented in Appendix C. The three composites and the total score may all be expressed as standard scores and percentile ranks. Teachers and parents are familiar and comfortable with percentile ranks as a method of ranking a student's performance. Salvia and Ysseldyke wrote that they "favor the use of percentile ranks. These unpretentious scores require the fewest assumptions for accurate interpretation" (1988, p. 93). However, because percentile ranks cannot be meaningfully added, subtracted, or averaged the way that standard scores can, the standard scores are suggested for use in comparing an individual child's composite and total scores (Hutchinson, 1996).

Score differences between males and females were studied during the analysis of the standardization data, and the results supported the construction of a single set of norms for males and females rather than separate norms by gender. The gender analyses are discussed in the section on construct validity later in this chapter.

RELIABILITY

As with any test, examiners wish to know if the results obtained from a single administration are reliable. Test reliability refers to the consistency with which the items on a test provide a stable score of the abilities being measured. Any discussion of reliability should begin with the observation that reliability, as much as validity, is meaningful only within the context in which the test is used. Thus, an examination of CSBS DP results must consider the conditions under which the test was administered, the similarity between the examinee and the sample with whom comparisons are to be made, and the type of decisions expected to follow from test results. In short, there are many aspects of reliability, and there are corresponding methods for estimating each. Four common methods are examined because they help answer four common questions:

- How does performance vary from item to item?
- How is the test's measurement error reflected when reporting performance?
- How does performance on the test change over time?
- How does performance on the test vary with the rater?

Internal Consistency

Internal consistency reliability coefficients express the degree to which the parts (in the case of CSBS DP, the individual items) in an evaluation instrument measure the same characteristic. Thus, an internal consistency coefficient helps to answer the first question: How much alike are the items on the test? The more that all items in a test measure the same variable, the higher we expect the internal consistency coefficient to be. Internal consistency coefficients are useful because they provide an estimate of the reliability of a test from a single administration and because they are not affected by changes in performance due to instruction or treatment; however, because internal consistency coefficients are influenced by a test's length and by the relative difficulties of the items in the test, one cannot always conclude from a high coefficient that all of the items in the test measure the same characteristic. Internal consistency coefficients (Cronbach's coefficient alpha) are reported by age intervals in Table 3.7 for the CSBS DP Infant-Toddler Checklist cluster, composite, and total scores. Internal consistency was estimated using Cronbach's coefficient alpha, which is based on the average split-half correlation coefficients among all of the individual items. These coefficients treat the individual items as polychotomous and should be regarded as conservative estimates of the internal consistency of the respective scores. The raw internal reliability coefficients of the composites and total for the Infant-Toddler Checklist are very high and indicate a high degree of internal consistency.

Standard Error of Measurement and Confidence Intervals

A major advantage of reliability coefficients is that they allow comparison between the reliability of different subtests or tests; however, these coefficients are not easily interpreted in terms of a particular child's score on a subtest or test. The standard error of measurement (SEM) employs the reliability coefficient to express the reliability of a subtest or test in terms

Table 3.7. Internal consistency reliability coefficients of the Infant-Toddler Checklist

Infant-Toddler Checklist							
						Coefficient alpha	
	n	*Mean*	*SD*	*Minimum*	*Maximum*	*Raw*	*Standardized*
Clusters							
Emotion and Eye Gaze	2188	7.04	1.00	1	8	.90	.96
Communication	2188	5.75	1.80	0	8	.89	.96
Gestures	2188	6.53	2.88	0	10	.88	.96
Sounds	2188	6.27	1.54	0	8	.89	.96
Words	2188	2.44	1.88	0	6	.89	.96
Understanding	2188	4.03	1.35	0	6	.89	.96
Object Use	2188	6.79	2.75	0	11	.88	.96
Composites							
Social	2188	19.31	4.91	2	26	.87	.95
Speech	2188	8.71	3.06	0	14	.88	.95
Symbolic	2188	10.82	3.85	0	17	.87	.95
Total	**2188**	**38.84**	**10.79**	**6**	**57**	**.93**	**.95**

of the obtained scores. That is, the SEM takes into account both the reliability of the test and the variability of performance, with the result expressed in the same unit of measurement as the obtained score. The formula used for calculating SEM is as follows:

$$\text{SEM} = \text{SD} \sqrt{(1\text{-Alpha})}$$

Thus, the SEM allows us to answer the second question: How is the test's measurement error reflected when reporting performance? Theoretically, the SEM describes a distance on either side of the child's true score—the score the child would receive if the test were perfectly reliable (i.e., if there were no measurement error associated with the test). However, because our only estimate of this theoretical true score is the child's obtained score, we use the SEM to build a range of scores around the obtained score. This range of scores around the obtained score permits us to express the child's performance in terms of an interval or band of error, rather than as a single, fixed score point with no indication of measurement error. We can also describe the degree of confidence associated with the band of error, and we can construct different confidence intervals for different levels of confidence. Of course, the larger the band of error the more confident we can be that the child's true score falls within the interval. To determine the bands of error, SEMs are multiplied by 1.0 for 68% confidence intervals, 1.65 for 90% confidence intervals, and 1.96 for 95% confidence intervals. Then, this number is added and subtracted from the score. For example, the 95% confidence interval is the score $\pm$ 1.96 $\times$ SEM.

SEMs are presented in Appendix C for the composite and total scores on the norms tables and are reported in standard score units along with 68%, 90%, and 95% confidence intervals. Confidence intervals can be easily calculated using the norms tables by adding and subtracting the weighted SEM from the standard score. The examiner should apply the bands of error to standard scores for the clusters, composites, and total scores to form the desired confidence interval.

The following is an example of calculating a confidence interval for a composite score. On the Social Composite of the Infant-Toddler Checklist, a 12-month-old child's raw score = 20. The standard score for this raw score = 11 (63rd percentile) and the SEM for the Social Composite standard score = 1.1.

68% Confidence Interval = 11 ± 1.1 = 9.9 to 12.1

90% Confidence Interval = 11 ± 1.8 = 9.2 to 12.8

95% Confidence Interval = 11 ± 2.1 = 8.9 to 13.1

This calculation gives you 68% confidence that this child's true score is somewhere between 10 and 12, and 95% confidence that it is between 9 and 13.

Test–Retest Stability

An important question for examiners using test results to monitor change is the third one noted in the list: How does performance on the test change over time? The term *stability* is often used to describe the consistency of test and retest results of subjects whose relative performance has not changed. Thus, to the extent that the test yields the same results for children, we consider it to be a stable, or reliable, measure. If, however, the relative standing of the children changes over time because of development or learning, we would expect the retest to yield results different from the test. Therefore, assessing stability requires us to compare test and retest scores where development or learning has had little or no effect on the child's relative standing in the group. Test–retest reliability coefficients describe the degree of relationship between scores obtained at two different times.

The test and retest scores of children who were retested within a year of the initial administration were compared to examine the stability of the CSBS DP scores over time. For the CSBS DP Infant-Toddler Checklist, retests were available for 167 children with a mean age of 13.2 months at the initial test ($SD = 3.7$) and a mean age of 17.3 months at retest ($SD = 3.8$). Table 3.8 reports a series of statistics for the children who had retests for the Infant-Toddler Checklist for both raw and standard composite and total scores. Table 3.8 lists the means and standard deviations of the test, retest, and differences between the mean scores for the two administrations. Pearson product moment correlation coefficients (r) were calculated to examine the relationship between the test and retest scores and are reported in Table 3.8 along with the significance level of the correlations. The Pearson correlation coefficient evaluates the strength of a relationship and ranges in value from -1 to $+1$. This coefficient indicates the degree that low or high scores on one variable (i.e., the extent that scores fall below or above the mean) tend to go with low or high scores on another variable (Tabachnick & Fidell, 2001). Correlation coefficients of .10, .30, and .50, regardless of sign, are interpreted as small, medium, and large coefficients,

Table 3.8. Test–retest reliabilities of raw and standard scores for the Infant-Toddler Checklist

		Test		Retest					Retest minus test		Effect size
	n	Mean	SD	Mean	SD	MD	r	p	t	p	
Raw scores											
Composites											
Social	167	17.81	5.84	20.73	4.48	2.92	.79	<.001	10.61	<.001	0.57***
Speech	167	7.72	2.95	9.62	3.01	1.90	.82	<.001	13.56	<.001	0.64**
Symbolic	167	10.00	3.96	12.68	3.46	2.68	.80	<.001	14.41	<.001	0.72**
Total	**167**	**35.53**	**11.68**	**43.04**	**9.75**	**7.50**	**.88**	**<.001**	**17.59**	**<.001**	**0.70****
Standard scores											
Composites											
Social	167	9.90	3.56	9.99	3.45	0.09	.72	<.001	0.44	ns	0.03
Speech	167	10.13	3.31	10.24	3.58	0.11	.67	<.001	0.52	ns	0.03
Symbolic	167	10.40	3.02	10.67	3.63	0.27	.65	<.001	1.22	ns	0.08
Total	**167**	**100.29**	**16.09**	**100.40**	**15.62**	**0.11**	**.86**	**<.001**	**0.17**	**ns**	**0.01**

*Small effect size; **Medium effect size; ***Large effect size; SD = standard deviation; MD = mean difference; ns = not significant.

respectively, in the behavioral sciences (Cohen, 1988). Eleven raw and standard score coefficients were significant and large, ranging from .65 to .88.

Differences between the test and retest scores were analyzed by calculating a t test of means for paired samples. The paired-samples t test evaluates whether the mean difference between the test and retest scores is significantly different from zero. The results of the t test and the level of significance are reported in Table 3.8. These results indicate that the mean retest raw scores were significantly greater than the mean initial test raw scores for all composite and total scores for the Infant-Toddler Checklist. In contrast, there were no significant differences between the standard scores from test to retest.

Effect sizes are also reported because they are useful for estimating the amount of growth over time and because they provide useful comparisons independent of sample size. The d statistic was computed as the effect size index by dividing the mean of the paired differences by the average of the standard deviations for the two samples. The average of the standard deviations was used because the variances for the two samples were not equal. When d equals 0, the distributions of the two samples are not different. As d diverges from 0, the effect size becomes larger. Regardless of sign, d values of .2, .5, and .8 represent small, medium, and large effect sizes, respectively (Cohen, 1988). The effect sizes for all of the raw scores are medium or large. In contrast, the effect sizes for none of the standard scores for the CSBS DP Infant-Toddler Checklist can be classified even as small, indicating that there are not appreciable differences in standard scores from test to retest. The effect sizes are consistent with the results of the t tests.

Taken together, these results indicate that the CSBS DP Infant-Toddler Checklist detects growth over short periods of time, based on changes in raw scores from test to retest. Furthermore, these results show that the Infant-Toddler Checklist produces relatively stable rankings of children, even when these children show significant improvement over a short period of time, based on the strong correlations of the raw and standard scores from test to retest and the stability of the standard scores from test to retest. The test–retest data provide additional evidence of high reliability for the CSBS DP.

Inter-rater Reliability

A fourth question addressing reliability is whether a child's performance is judged similarly by different raters, when judgments are required in scoring. This is not a concern for the Infant-Toddler Checklist because parents complete each item and the scores are simply tabulated.

VALIDITY

The concluding section of this chapter poses a series of questions about the validity of CSBS DP scores and decisions based on those scores. In simplest terms, validity is the extent to which judgments based on a test are accurate and appropriate for the intended purpose (Messick, 1989). Validity is generally regarded as evidence that a test measures what it purports to measure, and various types or sources of validity are distinguished by test makers and critics. Four major aspects of validity are reported: 1) content validity, or logical and theoretical support for the content and organization of items; 2) face validity, or the extent to which the test appears to measure particular behaviors; 3) construct validity, or statistical evidence that the test measures the construct or constructs intended by its authors; and 4) criterion validity, which includes evidence of agreement between scores on the test and scores on a criterion measure already regarded as valid.

Although these distinctions provide a useful framework for organizing evidence related to an instrument's validity, they should not be thought of as different kinds of validity, nor should they be thought of as substitutes for each other. We should not attribute validity to a test; validity is an issue of test use and the application of test information to interpretation and decision-making. As Messick noted, "Validity always refers to the degree to which empirical evidence and theoretical rationales support the adequacy and appropriateness of interpretations and actions based on test scores" (1989, p. 13). Ultimately, the validity of CSBS DP use will depend on how the results are applied to decisions about children's communication and symbolic behavior.

Content Validity

Judgments of content validity rely on a clear definition of the domain tested and the design of the test in relation to the domain, or what Messick called "the relevance and representativeness of the test items with respect to the domain" (1989, p. 17). The more clearly specified the rationale for the content, the more easily one can begin to assess the test's content validity. Evidence that the CSBS DP targets relevant domains of communication and symbolic behavior is provided in Chapter 2 of the CSBS DP Manual, which cites a rationale and relevant research literature that supports the instrument. The communication and symbolic behaviors measured are well documented in the literature as important skills that develop over the first 2 years of life. Statistical evidence supporting a developmental progression of behaviors measured is provided under the discussion of construct validity. The Infant-Toddler Checklist was designed to evaluate the same seven cluster areas derived from the research literature on prelinguistic predictors, reviewed in Chapter 1 of this manual. Statistical evidence supporting the relationship among the three components is provided under the discussion of criterion validity.

Face Validity

Face validity is the appearance of validity. That is, face validity is judged by appearance rather than by a detailed analysis of content as is done to establish content validity. For this reason, face validity has often been judged harshly and is often ignored. Researchers use the term ecological validity to describe the degree to which the setting of an experiment is similar to the setting to which the results are to be generalized. Recent proponents of authentic assessment argue that the ecological validity of an evaluation/ assessment is related to how the participants (e.g., a student and the teacher or parent and clinician) judge the appearance of a test. In these cases, at least, face validity may have to be considered an important aspect of an evaluation/assessment because the student and teacher or parent and clinician may show little commitment to the evaluation/assessment if they view its context and form as inauthentic or irrelevant.

For similar reasons, the CSBS DP procedures attempt to ensure the ecological validity of the information obtained by maximizing the role of the caregiver and using a naturalistic context. Bronfenbrenner has cautioned that our understanding of child development has been based on "the strange behavior of children in strange situations with strange adults for the briefest possible periods of time" (1979, p. viii). In the CSBS DP, the role of a caregiver as informant and participant and the use of sampling procedures with common toys and typical play activities are features that contribute to a more naturalistic context. This is usually not found with most tests made up of subtests with contrived tasks and independent items ordered by difficulty.

Construct Validity

Construct validity is statistical evidence that the test measures the construct or constructs it purports to measure. The statistical evidence can take the form of interpretable quantitative relationships between the test scores and other variables known to be related to the construct. Construct validity can also be shown through a study of the relationships among the various components of the test. In either case, the relationships of interest are those that could be predicted from the various elements in the test makers' theory or model of performance. Three types of construct validity data are presented in this section: developmental progression of scores, intercorrelations, and gender differences.

Developmental Progression of Scores

A test that measures communication and symbolic behaviors from 6 to 24 months of age should demonstrate growth and age differentiation because these skills show rapid development during the first 2 years of life. Table 3.9 reports the means and standard deviations of the raw scores for the Infant-Toddler Checklist composites and total by 1-month age intervals. The pattern of score increases on nearly all of the composite and total scores are consistent with growth on these aspects of communication and symbolic behaviors during this period of early development.

The developmental trends portrayed in Table 3.9 indicate that substantial growth is measured by the Infant-Toddler Checklist across the age

Table 3.9. Means and standard deviations (SD) of composite and total raw scores for the Infant-Toddler Checklist, by age in months

Age (months)	n	Composite						Total	
		Social		Speech		Symbolic			
		Mean	SD	Mean	SD	Mean	SD	Mean	SD
6	50	10.00	2.95	3.74	1.76	4.32	1.48	18.06	4.70
7	42	11.31	2.98	4.17	1.96	4.71	1.78	20.19	5.33
8	77	13.12	4.62	5.48	2.24	5.69	1.82	24.29	7.31
9	126	13.06	3.88	5.59	2.05	6.09	1.92	24.74	6.38
10	86	16.02	3.82	6.99	1.91	7.30	2.09	30.31	6.29
11	312	18.24	4.21	7.68	2.19	9.13	2.74	35.05	7.70
12	296	19.06	3.96	7.81	2.18	9.58	2.62	36.46	7.41
13	121	19.43	4.36	8.36	2.09	10.44	2.63	38.23	7.70
14	128	20.62	3.52	8.77	2.14	11.41	2.63	40.80	6.76
15	174	21.13	3.26	9.19	2.11	12.03	2.29	42.36	6.28
16	98	21.77	3.62	9.87	2.30	13.22	2.60	44.86	7.40
17	99	22.35	2.66	10.35	2.21	13.62	2.13	46.32	5.65
18	133	21.72	3.60	10.59	2.74	13.77	2.37	46.08	7.77
19	107	22.50	2.93	10.93	2.74	13.79	2.74	47.22	7.06
20	84	22.30	3.04	11.26	2.72	14.12	2.38	47.68	6.72
21	87	22.84	2.79	11.60	2.49	14.89	1.90	49.32	5.60
22	82	22.23	3.45	11.84	2.18	14.96	2.47	49.04	7.08
23	50	22.20	3.04	11.80	2.77	14.50	2.56	48.50	7.12
24	36	22.39	3.02	11.94	2.12	15.03	1.99	49.36	5.60
Total	2188								

span in the standardization sample. The composite raw scores increase at different rates across the age span represented in the standardization sample for the Infant-Toddler Checklist. The mean for the Social Composite is higher than either the Speech or Symbolic Composites at the younger age groups. Furthermore, the largest change on the Social Composite is evident for younger than 12 months for the Infant-Toddler Checklist, whereas that for the Speech and Symbolic Composites is evident for older than 12 months of age. The pattern of developmental growth in Table 3.9 indicates that the Social Composite and the clusters that comprise it measure skills that typically develop between 6 and 18 months of age, and the Speech and Symbolic Composites and corresponding clusters measure skills that continue to develop through 24 months of age.

Intercorrelations

An important issue in the use of the CSBS DP is the degree to which the individual items provide different information about the child's development. This issue was previously addressed under the topic of internal consistency with data in Table 3.7. Another approach to examining this issue is to study the intercorrelations among various subtests of a test, in this case the CSBS DP item composites and clusters. Traditionally, this approach is considered with construct validity. Table 3.10 presents a raw score intercorrelation matrix of composite scores for the Infant-Toddler

Table 3.10. Intercorrelations among composite raw scores of the Infant-Toddler Checklist for children in the standardized sample, by age

	n	Social	Speech
Ages 6–11 months			
Composites	693		
Speech		.65	
Symbolic		.69	.65
Ages 12–17 months			
Composites	916		
Speech		.54	
Symbolic		.62	.63
Ages 18–24 months			
Composites	579		
Speech		.51	
Symbolic		.57	.65
Ages 6–24 months			
Composites	2188		
Speech		.70	
Symbolic		.76	.78

$p<.001$
*$p<.01$
**$p<.05$
ns = not significant

Checklist, for 6-month age intervals and the entire sample. These correlations suggest that somewhat different skills or abilities are measured by each composite, although the different composites tend to demonstrate similar distributions of scores. The Speech and Symbolic Composites are generally more strongly related to each other than either one is to the Social Composite. These patterns are further supported by the intercorrelations among cluster scores. Table 3.11 presents a raw score intercorrelation matrix of cluster scores for the Infant-Toddler Checklist. Inspection of this table reveals a pattern of moderate correlations among most cluster scores when all ages are combined. When the 6-month age intervals are examined, stronger correlations are generally found among clusters within the same composites, and weaker correlations are found among clusters that are from different composites.

Gender Differences

The pattern of score increases by age may be contrasted with the pattern of score differences by gender. Whereas substantial changes in communication and symbolic behaviors may be predicted with increasing age during this period of early development, substantial differences between females and males would not be as predictable at these early ages. For this reason, a group of males and females were matched on age (to the tenth of a month) and race. Table 3.12 presents the comparison of the scores of the two matched groups on the Infant-Toddler Checklist with the result that

Table 3.11.   Intercorrelations among cluster raw scores of the Infant-Toddler Checklist for children in the standardization sample, by age

Clusters	Emotion	Communication	Gestures	Sounds	Words	Understanding
Ages 6–11 months						
n = 693						
Communication	.54					
Gestures	.44	.58				
Sounds	.37	.45	.51			
Words	.28	.38	.60	.45		
Understanding	.44	.48	.61	.45	.58	
Object Use	.34	.42	.65	.45	.59	.62
Ages 12–17 months						
n = 916						
Communication	.55					
Gestures	.42	.54				
Sounds	.38	.41	.42			
Words	.26	.32	.45	.49		
Understanding	.43	.42	.52	.44	.60	
Object Use	.39	.41	.53	.41	.50	.56
Ages 18–24 months						
n = 579						
Communication	.50					
Gestures	.46	.53				
Sounds	.34	.40	.47			
Words	.27	.36	.42	.65		
Understanding	.41	.40	.44	.54	.59	
Object Use	.34	.42	.46	.49	.51	.52
Ages 6–24 months						
n = 2188						
Communication	.57					
Gestures	.47	.66				
Sounds	.41	.52	.59			
Words	.32	.49	.65	.60		
Understanding	.46	.57	.69	.58	.73	
Object Use	.40	.56	.73	.57	.72	.74

$p<.001$
*$p<.01$
**$p<.05$
ns = not significant

no substantial differences were found on almost all of the clusters. Table 3.12 lists the means and standard deviations of females and males, the differences between the mean scores for the two groups, the results of a *t* test for paired samples, and the effect size of each difference. This statistical analysis is similar to that on test–retest stability reported previously in the chapter in the section on reliability.

For the CSBS DP Infant-Toddler Checklist, none of the *t* tests of differences were significant for the composite scores and the total score. The Gesture Cluster for the Infant-Toddler Checklist reached the .05 level-of-significance; however, norms are presented only for composite scores for the Infant-Toddler Checklist, and the Social Composite was not significantly different for females and males. None of the cluster, composite, or

Table 3.12. Comparisons of raw scores for the Infant-Toddler Checklist for matched pairs of females and males in the standardized sample

n = 253 pairs	Female		Male		Female minus male			
	Mean	SD	Mean	SD	MD	t	p	Effect size
Clusters								
Emotion and								
Eye Gaze	7.05	1.00	6.92	0.96	0.13	1.50	ns	0.13
Communication	5.64	1.89	5.64	1.77	0.00	−0.02	ns	0.00
Gestures	6.60	3.11	6.03	2.99	0.57	2.08	<.05	0.19
Sounds	6.60	1.56	6.09	1.63	0.21	1.48	ns	0.13
Words	2.56	2.04	2.32	1.93	0.24	1.37	ns	0.12
Understanding	4.04	1.42	3.87	1.39	0.17	1.36	ns	0.12
Object Use	6.91	3.07	6.56	2.63	0.35	1.37	ns	0.12
Composites								
Social	19.28	5.24	18.59	4.98	0.69	1.52	ns	0.14
Speech	8.86	3.33	8.41	3.22	0.45	1.55	ns	0.14
Symbolic	10.94	4.25	10.42	3.76	0.52	1.45	ns	0.13
Total	**39.08**	**11.85**	**37.42**	**10.96**	**1.66**	**1.64**	**ns**	**0.15**

MD = mean difference; ns = not significant.

total scores for the Infant-Toddler Checklist had effect sizes that would be considered small, medium, or large. These data lend support to the use of one set of norms for both males and females; however, it is noteworthy that all of the differences were in the direction of females scoring higher, although the differences were negligible or small.

Criterion Validity

Because there are so few measures designed specifically to assess the communicative and symbolic behavior of children younger than 24 months of age, criterion validity studies of the CSBS DP are necessarily limited; however, a series of studies were conducted to examine both concurrent and predictive validity, which are aspects of criterion validity using standardized measures of language and related abilities. Concurrent validity is evidence that scores on an instrument accurately indicate how subjects would be classified by an independent criterion administered at the same point in time, whereas predictive validity is evidence that scores on an instrument accurately predict how subjects would be classified by an independent criterion administered at a time in the future. For the CSBS DP, both concurrent and predictive validity address practical questions because they relate to how useful the scores may be in identifying children at risk for potential delays or disorders.

Concurrent Validity

The concurrent validity of the Infant-Toddler Checklist was evaluated by comparing standard scores between the Infant-Toddler Checklist and the other two components of the CSBS DP—the Caregiver Questionnaire and the Behavior Sample. Subjects were drawn from children in the standardization sample and a pool of about 50 children with communication and language delays. Since the CSBS DP will be used with children who have developmental delays, we felt that it was important to include them in the studies of concurrent validity. Children were selected for this study if they had completed the Infant-Toddler Checklist and one of the other components at the same age (plus or minus 3 months). The relationship among the Infant-Toddler Checklist, Caregiver Questionnaire, and Behavior Sample was examined by calculating Pearson correlation coefficients on pairs of standard scores obtained from the same children.

The correlation coefficients for the composite and total standard scores on the Infant-Toddler Checklist and Caregiver Questionnaire, Caregiver Questionnaire and Behavior Sample, and the Infant-Toddler Checklist and Behavior Sample are presented in Table 3.13.

Large, significant correlations were observed among all of the total scores, and moderate or large, significant correlations were observed among all of the composites. Patterns of the correlations are noteworthy. The strongest correlations were observed between the Infant-Toddler Checklist and the Caregiver Questionnaire, which are both parent report measures. Very similar correlations were found between the Caregiver Questionnaire and the Behavior Sample and between the Infant-Toddler Checklist and the Behavior Sample. In comparing across composites, the strongest correlations were generally observed for the Speech Composite,

Table 3.13.   Correlations and total standard scores for the Infant-Toddler Checklist (ITC), Caregiver Questionnaire (CQ), and Behavior Sample (BS) administered within 3 months, by age

	n	ITC & CQ	n	CQ & BS	n	ITC & BS
Ages 6–11 months						
Composites	77					
Social		.50				
Speech		.54				
Symbolic		.53				
Total		**.56**				
Ages 12–17 months						
Composites	215		123		100	
Social		.77		.44		.47
Speech		.74		.63		.54
Symbolic		.71		.62		.53
Total		**.80**		**.66**		**.62**
Ages 18–24 months						
Composites	202		140		84	
Social		.73		.44		.38
Speech		.84		.76		.74
Symbolic		.79		.58		.57
Total		**.88**		**.71**		**.68**

$p<.001$
*$p<.01$
**$p<.05$
ns = not significant

followed by the Symbolic Composite. The strongest correlations were also generally observed for the oldest age group (18–24 months).

These findings support the validity of these parent report tools as a measure of early communication and symbolic abilities. The Infant-Toddler Checklist, which is a brief parent report tool, had a very strong correlation with the Caregiver Questionnaire, a more in-depth parent report tool. Furthermore, there was a strong relationship between children's standard scores on the parent report tools (i.e., Infant–Toddler Checklist and Caregiver Questionnaire) and those based on the face-to-face evaluation of the child (i.e., Behavior Sample).

Predictive Validity

The predictive validity of the CSBS DP Infant-Toddler Checklist was evaluated by comparing the standard scores with children's outcomes on standardized testing at 2 and 3 years of age. The Mullen Scales of Early Learning (Mullen, 1995), which measures gross motor, fine motor, visual recognition, receptive language, and expressive language and provides an Early Learning Composite of the four cognitive scales (i.e., excluding gross motor), was used for the follow-up standardized testing. This measure was selected because it has good psychometric features, provides a cognitive composite, and also provides separate scores for receptive and expressive language. Subjects were drawn from children in the standardization sample and a pool of about 60 children at risk for communication and language delays. Children at risk were defined as those who performed in the bottom 10th percentile based on the CSBS DP. These children were recruited from health care and child care agencies who administered the Infant-Toddler Checklist, and their families were invited to complete the Caregiver Questionnaire and Behavior Sample. About 120 typical children were randomly selected from the standardization sample in the Tallahassee region based on scores above the 10th percentile on the CSBS DP. All of these families were invited to bring their children in for follow-up standardized testing just after their second birthday and again after their third birthday.

The relationship between the Infant-Toddler Checklist and the Mullen Scales was examined by calculating Pearson correlation coefficients on pairs of standard scores obtained from the same children. The Receptive Language Scale, Expressive Language Scale, and Learning Composite of the Mullen Scales and the Social, Speech, and Symbolic Composites and the Total of the Infant-Toddler Checklist were used for this analysis. The mean and standard deviation of the test scores and the children's age at administration and the correlation coefficients (r) between components are presented in Table 3.14 for the 2-year-old follow-up testing and Table 3.15 for the 3-year-old follow-up testing.

Moderate to large, significant correlations were observed among all of the scores both at 2- and 3-year-old follow-up testing. Patterns of the correlations are noteworthy. In comparing across composites, the strongest correlations were generally observed between the CSBS DP Speech Composite and the Expressive Language Scale of the Mullen Scales and

Table 3.14. Correlations of standard scores for the Infant-Toddler Checklist with the Mullen Scales of Early Learning administered at 2 years

			Mullen Scales of Early Learning									
			Receptive language			Expressive language			Learning composite			Age (months)	
n = 192	Mean	SD	Mean	SD	r	Mean	SD	r	Mean	SD	r	Mean	SD
Infant-Toddler Checklist													
Composites			50.9	15.0		46.5	15.1		99.6	24.2		25.2	1.7
Social	9.1	3.3			.48			.43			.48		
Speech	8.5	3.1			.39			.50			.43		
Symbolic	9.4	3.2			.54			.41			.58		
Total	93.4	15.9			.54			.51			.57		
Age (months)	14.0	4.2											

Note: Mullen Scales scores for the Receptive and Expressive Language Scales are T scores (M = 50, SD = 10) and for the Learning Composite are standard scores (M = 100, SD = 15). CSBS DP scores are standard scores for the composites (M = 10, SD = 3) and Total (M = 100, SD = 15).

Table 3.15. Correlations of standard scores for the Infant-Toddler Checklist with the Mullen Scales of Early Learning administered at 3 years

			Mullen Scales of Early Learning										
			Receptive language			Expressive language			Learning composite			Age (months)	
n = 92	Mean	SD	Mean	SD	r	Mean	SD	r	Mean	SD	r	Mean	SD
Infant-Toddler Checklist													
Composites			49.6	12.1		52.0	13.1		106.3	24.4		37.9	2.2
Social	8.5	3.3			.33			.38			.40		
Speech	8.2	3.3			.28*			.39			.35		
Symbolic	9.0	3.3			.49			.56			.56		
Total	90.5	16.4			.40			.49			.48		
Age (months)	16.1	4.0											

Note: Mullen Scales scores for the Receptive and Expressive Language Scales are T scores (M = 50, SD = 10) and for the Learning Composite are standard scores (M = 100, SD = 15). CSBS DP scores are standard scores for the composites (M = 10, SD = 3) and Total (M = 100, SD = 15).
p <.001 unless otherwise noted
*p <.01

between the CSBS DP Symbolic Composite and the Receptive Language Scale of the Mullen Scales. The strongest correlations were generally observed between the Learning Composite of the Mullen Scales and the Total of the CSBS DP. The correlations were larger at the 2-year-old follow-up testing than at the 3-year-old follow-up testing, but the relationships continued to be significant at the 3-year-old follow-up testing.

Using the same data, predictive validity was also evaluated by comparing the classification of the child's performance based on the Infant-Toddler Checklist with the classification of performance based on the follow-up standardized testing at 2 and 3 years of age. First, we had to decide our criteria for being at risk on the CSBS DP and failing the follow-up testing. Many tests and state eligibility criteria use the criteria of either 2 or 1.5 standard deviations below the mean as a cutoff, which corresponds with the 2nd and 7th percentiles, respectively. However, we chose 1.25 standard deviations below the mean, which corresponds with the 10th percentile, because 10%–15% of school-age children have developmental disabilities that require special education, and our goal is to improve early identification of these children. Children were classified as at risk if they performed in the bottom 10th percentile (i.e., a standard score at or below 6 on the composites and 81 on the total).

For the Infant-Toddler Checklist, the criterion for at risk was set at performance in the bottom 10th percentile for the Social or Symbolic Composite or Total. Children who were in the bottom 10th percentile on only the Speech Composite were not considered at risk because this led to the inclusion of too many late talkers who cleared up; if they also scored low on either the Social or Symbolic Composite, they were more likely to have persisting problems.

At follow-up testing, children were classified as having failed the Mullen Scales if they performed in the bottom 10th percentile on at least two of the five scales (i.e., Gross Motor, Visual Reception, Fine Motor, Receptive Language, and Expressive Language) or on the Learning Composite or in the bottom 2nd percentile on at least one of the five scales.

Agreement between classifications on the Infant-Toddler Checklist and the 2- and 3-year-old follow-up standardized testing are presented in two-way contingency tables in Table 3.16. The following agreement proportions were calculated for the Infant-Toddler Checklist to evaluate validity and are reported in Table 3.16:

- True positives—the proportion of children identified as at risk (i.e., receiving a positive screen or evaluation result) who failed the follow-up testing; also called sensitivity

- True negatives—the proportion of children identified as no risk (i.e., receiving a negative screen or evaluation result) who passed the follow-up testing; also called specificity

- False positives—the proportion of children identified as at risk (i.e., receiving a positive screen or evaluation result) who passed the follow-up testing

Table 3.16. Contingency table for the CSBS DP with the Mullen Scales of Early Learning administered at 2 and 3 years of age

	Fail	Pass	
Identified at risk	35	26	61
No risk	11	120	131
	46	146	192

2-year-old follow-up

True positives (Sensitivity)	76.1%
True negatives (Specificity)	82.2%
False positives	17.8%
False negatives	23.9%
Percent agreement	80.7%
Overreferral	13.5%
Underreferral	5.7%
Positive predictive value	57.4%
Negative predictive value	91.6%

	Fail	Pass	
Identified at risk	16	20	36
No risk	3	53	56
	19	73	92

3-year-old follow-up

True positives (Sensitivity)	84.2%
True negatives (Specificity)	72.6%
False positives	27.4%
False negatives	15.8%
Percent agreement	75.0%
Overreferral	21.7%
Underreferral	3.3%
Positve predictive value	44.4%
Negative predictive value	94.6%

- False negatives—the proportion of children identified as no risk (i.e., receiving a negative screen or evaluation result) who failed the follow-up testing

- Percent agreement—the proportion of children correctly identified as either at risk or no risk, based on passing or failing the follow-up testing, respectively

- Overreferral—the proportion of children incorrectly identified as at risk out of the total number of children screened or evaluated

- Underreferral—the proportion of children incorrectly identified as no risk out of the total number of children screened or evaluated

- Positive predictive value—the proportion of children identified as at risk who failed the follow-up testing out of the total number of children identified as at risk.

- Negative predictive value—the proportion of children identified as no risk who pass the follow-up testing out of the total number of children identified as no risk.

These results provide good evidence for the predictive validity of the CSBS DP Infant-Toddler Checklist. Agreement proportions for the Infant-Toddler Checklist indicate good validity for a brief screening measure. These agreement proportions are based on criterion testing that ranges from 4–11 months later at the 2-year-old follow-up testing and 18–22 months later at the 3-year-old follow-up testing. This is particularly noteworthy because the agreement proportions are comparable or better in comparison with what other instruments have documented for concurrent validity (i.e., based on comparison with other measures gathered at the same time) with infants and toddlers.

In conclusion, these validation studies demonstrate that the Infant-Toddler Checklist is effective at screening early prelinguistic communication skills and predicting a child's relative performance on measures 1–2 years later. These findings strongly support the predictive validity of the CSBS DP Infant-Toddler Checklist and the use of a collection of prelinguistic measures, rather than the use of words alone, to improve the accuracy of early identification of very young children. However, it is important to be aware of the inaccuracy of any evaluation tool. That is, on parent report measures, a small proportion of parents overestimate or underestimate their children's abilities. On the face-to-face evaluation, a small proportion of children perform below their potential or the measure does not detect a small proportion of children who will have later learning problems. It is for this reason that we designed the CSBS DP to utilize multiple sources of information and that we strongly recommend using a combination of parent report and face-to-face evaluation procedures with very young children.

INTERPRETING RESULTS 4

This chapter describes how to interpret the results for the CSBS DP Infant-Toddler Checklist. The first part of this chapter describes general issues for interpreting results. The last part of the chapter addresses screening decisions based on the Checklist and provides guidelines for writing a screening report.

GENERAL ISSUES FOR INTERPRETING THE CSBS DP INFANT-TODDLER CHECKLIST

The reliability and validity findings reported in Chapter 3 support the use of the Infant-Toddler Checklist as a screening tool with children 6–24 months of age. One advantage of the Infant-Toddler Checklist is that it maximizes the role of the family in screening by utilizing a cost-efficient parent report tool, which reflects family-centered practices, as mandated for infants and toddlers by the Individuals with Disabilities Education (IDEA) Act Amendments of 1997 (PL 105-17). Another advantage of the Infant-Toddler Checklist is that standard scores and percentiles are available, whereas most screening tools report only pass/fail cutoff scores. Normative scores allow service providers to decide the cutoff based on state eligibility requirements and to monitor more carefully children who fall between the 10th and 25th percentiles. Eligibility criteria for early intervention services through Part C of IDEA vary from state to state, ranging from 1 to 2 standard deviations below the mean. However, if we are going to improve early identification of children with developmental disabilities, we need to use eligibility criteria that will catch a sensible proportion of children. Because 10%–15% of school-age children have disabilities, we recommend a cutoff of at least 1.25 SD below the mean, particularly for screening, which corresponds to the bottom 10th percentile. This will allow earlier identification of the majority of children who will require special education at school age. By setting the cutoff at 2 standard deviations below the mean, which corresponds to the bottom 2nd percentile, we will continue to miss most of the children who will require special education when they get to school age.

The accuracy and effectiveness of parent report compared to face-to-face evaluation is difficult to disentangle with very young children.

There are advantages and limitations of both evaluation methods. Parent report can be inaccurate if parents over- or under-estimate their children's abilities. The strength of the relationship between our parent report tools and the face-to-face evaluation reported in Chapter 3 suggests a moderate to high degree of accuracy, similar to the research findings with other parent report tools (Fenson et al., 1993; Rescorla & Alley, 2001; Squires, Potter, & Bricker, 1999). However, there is still a degree of inaccuracy with parent report. Therefore, it is important to use a parent report tool with caution and sound clinical judgment so that parents are not needlessly concerned. The three components of the CSBS DP can be used in combination so that a clinical decision is based on both parent report and a face-to-face evaluation.

One possible way to increase the accuracy of parent report is to use more than one parent report tool. The Ages & Stages Questionnaires (ASQ, Squires et al., 1999) is a widely used child-monitoring system, which, like the CSBS DP Infant-Toddler Checklist, uses parent report as a method to screen young children. The ASQ has questionnaires from 4 months to 48 months linked to specific ages (e.g., 12-month questionnaire). Each questionnaire includes 6 questions in five domains and has pass/fail cutoff points. We recommend using the ASQ along with the CSBS DP Infant-Toddler Checklist or follow-up CSBS DP Caregiver Questionnaire because they provide complementary information.

Parent report is ineffective if parents do not complete and return the evaluation tool. In research on parent report tools, a large percentage of parents do not return questionnaires received in the mail, ranging from 64% when not contacted ahead (Fenson, et al., 1993) to 25%–40% when contacted ahead and families agreed to return the questionnaires (Fenson et al., 1993; Rescorla & Alley, 2001; Wetherby, Allen, Cleary, Kublin, & Goldstein, in press). Therefore, when using parent report for screening and evaluation, it is important to plan follow-up methods if questionnaires are mailed to families. We find the Checklist to be most effective if it can be completed by families when given out by staff at a healthcare or childcare facility, rather than asking the family to return the checklist in the mail.

Although parents may over- or underestimate their child's abilities with parent report tools, it is also challenging to secure accurate measures of abilities in very young children based on face-to-face evaluations. Many factors may influence children's performance, including attention, interest, fatigue, comfort level, and experience being in unfamiliar settings. The naturalistic sampling procedures of the CSBS DP Behavior Sample were designed to put the child and parent at ease and encourage communication. Having the parent present and participating during the Behavior Sample should increase the likelihood of gathering a representative sample. This also provides a context to build consensus with the family about the child's strengths and weaknesses. A face-to-face evaluation may be limited in effectiveness because families may not agree to participate in an evaluation or may not show up for a scheduled evaluation. We recommend using a combination of parent report and face-to-face evaluation to offer families both methods. For families who choose to participate in both, this provides the opportunity to look for a convergence of findings from multiple sources of information, and if the findings are discrepant, to explore reasons why they are so.

Socioeconomic Class

A limitation of the normative sample for the CSBS DP is the under-representation of families from lower socioeconomic (SES) classes. We had good success in having families from minority races complete the Checklist, but have only a small proportion of families from lower SES participate in the normative sample. The age and education level of the families participating in the normative sample are very similar to normative samples with other standardized evaluation tools for young children (e.g., Fenson, et al., 1993; Mullen, 1995).

Extreme caution is needed in using the Infant-Toddler Checklist and other screening and evaluation tools with families from low SES classes, if they are not well represented in the normative sample. In studies of social class with the MacArthur Child Development Inventory (CDI) (Fenson et al., 1992), there were significant differences in word comprehension on the CDI/Words and Gestures and in vocabulary production on the CDI/Words and Sentences for children 20 months of age and younger. With the CDI there was a tendency for lower-SES parents to check more items on the inventories than parents of higher SES. These findings suggest that parents with less education may overestimate their children's language abilities and that parents with more education may underestimate their children's language abilities. We recommend that when using the Infant-Toddler Checklist with a parent who has less than a high school education, a service provider should go over the information in a face-to-face meeting with the parent to ensure that the parent understands the questions. It is important to consider ways to offer developmental screening and evaluation so that a greater number of families from diverse cultures and SES classes will participate.

Ceiling and Floor Effects

As commonly found with standardized tools, there are ceiling and floor effects with the components of the CSBS DP. It is important for the evaluator to be aware of these and to use this information in interpreting results. A *ceiling effect* is when a large proportion of children in a normative age group is at ceiling or achieving the maximum possible score. A *floor effect* is when a large proportion of children in a normative age group is at floor or achieving the minimum possible score. A ceiling or floor effect is evident to a small extent for the total and composite scores and to a greater extent for some of the clusters. The norms tables for each component reveal where ceiling and floor effects exist.

A *ceiling effect* is evident if the highest possible raw score spans across several standard scores (and corresponding percentiles) for a particular age.

In creating the norms tables, if a raw score fell across several different standard scores, we assigned the raw score to the highest one. Thus, the cells in the norms table are blank if there were repeated raw scores. Refer to the Checklist norms table. For example, at 24 months, a child who earned a raw score of 26 on the Social Composite of the Checklist has a standard score ranging from 13 to 17 and percentile ranging from 84 to 99, and would be assigned a 17 standard score and 99th percentile because it is the highest score and a conservative estimate of this child's relative standing in the group. But that child could be functioning as low as the 84th percentile.

Continue to refer to the Checklist norms table to identify ceiling effects. For the Social Composite of the Checklist, there is a very slight ceiling effect beginning at 12 months of age, which becomes more prominent at 21 months. What this means is that the Checklist is not differentiating between children who perform between the 84th and 99th percentile at 24 months. For the Speech and Symbolic Composites and the Total there is also a very slight ceiling effect beginning at about 14 months of age, which becomes more prominent at 21 months. The largest ceiling effect found on the Checklist is on the Speech and Symbolic Composites at 22–24 months of age. The highest possible score of 14 on the Speech Composite and 17 on the Symbolic Composite corresponds to a standard score ranging from 12 to 17 and percentile ranging from 75 to 99.

For clinical use of the Infant-Toddler Checklist, a ceiling effect is not problematic because we are trying to be precise in identifying children who fall at the bottom end of the normative tables, rather than the top end. In fact, it can offer more confidence in expectations that children should be able to perform the skills that are being measured. When a large ceiling effect exists, caution should be taken in interpreting a child's score as above average versus average. Other tools that are more precise measures of language at the older age range should be used in combination with the Infant-Toddler Checklist (e.g., the Language Development Survey, Rescorla, 1989). A ceiling effect may be problematic for research studies using correlational analyses because there will be a restricted range where there is a ceiling effect. However, the extent of the ceiling effect was not problematic for the studies that we have conducted and reported in this manual. Using the Composites instead of the Clusters will reduce the extent of the ceiling effect.

A *floor effect* is evident if the lowest possible score spans across several standard scores (and corresponding percentiles) for a particular age. As noted above, in creating the norms tables, if a raw score fell across several different standard scores, we assigned the raw score to the highest one, which may overestimate an individual child's relative performance. Floor effects are not evident on the Checklist norms.

Children Older than 24 Months of Age

The norms for the Infant-Toddler Checklist only go through 24 months of age. The Infant-Toddler Checklist can be used with children older than 24 months of age as long as they are functioning below a 24-month age level. A child older than 24 months of age can be compared to the oldest age group (i.e., 24 months for the Infant-Toddler Checklist). However, the evaluator needs to be very careful in interpreting and reporting standard scores and percentiles. If any of the child's scores fall above the concern range (i.e., above the 10th percentile), you cannot be confident that the child is performing as expected for his or her age because we do not know whether children older than 24 months would score even higher on these measures. In other words, the standard scores and percentiles may be over-estimating the child's true performance because you are comparing that child to a younger normative group.

For example, if you use the Checklist with a 26-month-old child and the child scores in the 16th percentile or higher on all composites, you should *not* send a report indicating that the child is performing as expected for his or her age. Rather, you need to inform the parents that the child is too old to use the norms for this tool. If that child scores at the 9th percentile, it would be appropriate to refer that child for an evaluation. However, it is important to only report that the child is performing in the bottom 10th percentile and not report the specific percentile because that child may actually be performing lower than the 9th percentile when compared to same-age children. Keep in mind that if the child is performing in the bottom 10th percentile, we recommend that you not report the specific percentile to parents even for children younger than 24 months (see sample reports in next section).

Screening Decisions Based on the Infant-Toddler Checklist

The Infant-Toddler Checklist is a first step in routine developmental screening for children 6–24 months of age to decide if a developmental evaluation is needed. The scoring decisions for the Checklist are provided in Chapter 2 and Appendix B. A service provider may use the Checklist without using the other components of the CSBS DP. If a child is referred for a developmental evaluation using more traditional evaluation tools that measure receptive and expressive language as a follow-up to the Checklist, it is possible that there will not be agreement because the Checklist is measuring different skills. Because the CSBS DP measures social and symbolic aspects of communication and language development, it may identify children as at risk who may perform better on more traditional tests that only measure vocabulary or structural aspects of language. This can be confusing to families so it is important that users of the Checklist understand the domains that it measures.

It is recommended that the Checklist be used to monitor development about every 3 months between 6 and 24 months. Because it is based on parent report, it is possible for the caregiver to overestimate or underestimate the child's abilities. Therefore, this tool should be used along with a brief observation of the child by a health care or child care service provider. The Checklist should only be used to decide that further information or a developmental evaluation is needed. Caution should be taken not to alarm parents. We find that many parents already have concerns about their child, especially as their child is approaching about 18 months of age and is behind in language development. As noted above, the early intervention literature emphasizes the notion of multiple risk factors, and therefore a child's scores on this Checklist need to be considered in relation to other known biological or environmental risk factors. Clinical judgment should be used in making decisions about the need for further evaluation with the standard scores as guidelines. Remember that the Checklist is not meant for a developmental or diagnostic evaluation and should not be used to determine if a child has a developmental delay or to make a differential diagnosis.

Guidelines for Reporting the Infant-Toddler Checklist Results

We have developed two report formats for the CSBS DP Infant-Toddler Checklist. One is the Infant-Toddler Checklist: Screening Report, which includes the child's raw scores, standard scores, and percentiles ranks and is placed in the child's health record. The other is a letter to parents that summarizes the recommendation based on the Infant-Toddler Checklist results, which should be sent within 1 week of receiving the Checklist. The letter to parents does not include scores but briefly explains what the Checklist measures, whether a developmental evaluation is recommended, and if so, why this evaluation is important. We have developed three different versions of the letter to parents based on the recommendation made. The first letter, included in Figure 4.1, is for children who perform in the no concern range on all three composites and indicates that the child is currently communicating as expected for his or her age and that the child should be monitored with another checklist in 3 months. The second letter, included in Figure 4.2 , is for children who perform in the concern range on the Speech Composite only for the first time and recommends that the child should be monitored with another checklist in 3 months. The third letter, included in Figure 4.3, is for children who perform in the concern range on the Social and/or Symbolic Composite and recommends referring the child for a developmental evaluation.

An example of the Infant-Toddler Checklist: Screening Report and the letter to parents for a sample child, Casey Smith, is included in Figure 4.4. The information reported by Casey's mother on the Infant-Toddler Checklist indicates that he is in the concern range on the Speech and Symbolic Composites, and therefore, a developmental evaluation is recommended. The wording of these reports should be used as a model for reporting information from the Infant-Toddler Checklist. These reports can be generated and printed with the **Infant-Toddler Checklist and Easy-Score** software program. As explained in Chapter 2, the Easy-Score program generates a Screening Report with standard scores, percentile ranks, and concern indicated if the child's scores fall more than 1.25 standard deviations below the mean. The Easy-Score program allows the user to select one of the three letters for the parents based on the child's pattern of scores and recommendation made.

Re: (CSBS DP) Infant-Toddler Checklist

Child's name: ─────────────────────

Date of birth: ─────────────────────

Date Checklist completed: ──────────────

Chronological age (in months): ──────────

Referral recommended: No

Dear (parent's name):

Thank you for taking the time to complete the *Infant-Toddler Checklist*. The Checklist was used to screen your child's ability to communicate using eye gaze, gestures, sounds, or words and to play with toys.

Based on the information you provided on the Checklist, your child is currently communicating as expected for his or her age. Because new skills are emerging each month, it is important to monitor (child's name)'s development, and we would like you to complete the Checklist again in about 3 months.

We will contact you at the appropriate time to provide you with a Checklist. If you have any questions or concerns about your child's development, please feel free to call us.

We look forward to assisting you.

Sincerely,

(Examiner's name)

Figure 4.1.   Letter to parents with referral not recommended.

Re: (CSBS DP) Infant-Toddler Checklist

Child's name: _____

Date of birth: _____

Date Checklist completed: _____

Chronological age (in months): _____

Referral recommended: Not Yet

Dear (parent's name):

Thank you for taking the time to complete the *Infant-Toddler Checklist*. The Checklist was used to screen your child's ability to communicate using eye gaze, gestures, sounds, or words and to play with toys.

Based on the information you provided on the Checklist, we are recommending that your child's development be monitored so we can see how (child's name)'s skills are emerging. We would like you to complete the Checklist again in about 3 months.

We will contact you at the appropriate time to provide you with a Checklist. If you have any questions or concerns about your child's development, please feel free to call us.

We look forward to assisting you.

Sincerely,

(Examiner's name)

Figure 4.2.   Letter to parents with referral not yet recommended.

Re: (CSBS DP) **Infant-Toddler Checklist**

Child's name: _____

Date of birth: _____

Date Checklist completed: _____

Chronological age (in months): _____

Referral recommended: Yes

Dear (parent's name):

Thank you for taking the time to complete the *Infant-Toddler Checklist*. The Checklist was used to screen (child's name)'s ability to communicate using eye gaze, gestures, sounds, or words and to play with toys.

Based on the information you provided on the Checklist, we are recommending that (child's name) be referred for a developmental evaluation. Please call our office so we can help make these arrangements.

The Checklist does not conclusively determine if your child has a problem in development, but indicates whether further evaluation or follow-up is needed. A more thorough developmental evaluation can determine if (child's name) has a communication delay. If needed, we will provide information for planning the next steps to support you and your child. Children who have early communication delays may have difficulties in other areas of development. It is important to catch communication problems in young children as early as possible, as early intervention services may remediate or lessen the impact of communication problems and help you support your child's development.

We look forward to assisting you.

Sincerely,

(Examiner's name)

Figure 4.3.   Letter to parents with referral recommended.

Re: (CSBS DP) **Infant-Toddler Checklist**

Child's name: <u>Casey Smith</u>

Date of birth: <u>May 17, 2000</u>

Date Checklist completed: <u>February 24, 2002</u>

Chronological age (in months): <u>20 months</u>

Referral recommended: Yes

Dear Ms. Smith:

Thank you for taking the time to complete the *Infant-Toddler Checklist*. The Checklist was used to screen Casey's ability to communicate using eye gaze, gestures, sounds, or words and to play with toys.

Based on the information you provided on the Checklist, we are recommending that Casey be referred for a developmental evaluation. Please call our office so we can help make these arrangements.

The Checklist does not conclusively determine if your child has a problem in development but indicates whether further evaluation or follow-up is needed. A more thorough developmental evaluation can determine if Casey has a communication delay. If needed, we will provide information for planning the next steps to support you and your child. Children who have early communication delays may have difficulties in other areas of development. It is important to catch communication problems in young children as early as possible, as early intervention services may remediate or lessen the impact of communication problems and help you support your child's development.

We look forward to assisting you.

Sincerely,

Jane Miller, M.S., CCC-SLP

Figure 4.4.   Letter to parents for Casey.

SUMMARY

There is wide variation in the age that children begin talking and the rate that children learn to talk. This makes it difficult to decide when to be concerned if a child is not talking. The sounds and gestures children use to communicate and the ability to understand words and to play with objects provide important clues about the development of language. Families are often the first to raise concerns about their child's development. Concerns raised by the majority of families are warranted (Glascoe, 1999), and therefore, it is very important to conduct a developmental screening for any child whose family has any concern about his or her development. Some families have concerns about their child, but their child is developing typically. It is important to reassure those families and provide information about developmental milestones and their child's development. Some infants and toddlers are delayed but families are not yet concerned. It can be difficult for parents to learn that their child is not developing as expected. It is important not to alarm families, in light of the degree of inaccuracy of developmental screenings, and to offer support as concerns are raised. It can be confusing to families if one professional tells them that their child is doing fine and another indicates concern, and therefore, it is important to coordinate efforts for interdisciplinary evaluations of young children.

The CSBS DP was designed for screening and evaluation of children in the early stages of communication development. Using a parent report tool, such as the CSBS DP Infant-Toddler Checklist, minimizes the time required of healthcare providers, maximizes the role of the family, and provides reasonably accurate information about whether to refer a child for a developmental evaluation. The CSBS DP Caregiver Questionnaire and Behavior Sample offer a follow-up evaluation to the Infant-Toddler Checklist utilizing multiple sources of information to build consensus with the family on whether the child has a developmental delay. The CSBS DP offers a clinical tool that supports the use of prelinguistic predictors to improve early identification and maximizes the role of the family in the screening and evaluation process. It should be used with sound clinical judgment to decide whether a child needs further evaluation and/or early intervention and to monitor a child's growth in early communication development.

REFERENCES

Angoff, W.H. (1971). Scales, norms, and equivalent scores. In R.L. Thorndike (Ed.), *Educational measurement* (2nd ed.). Washington, DC: American Council on Education.

Baker, L. & Cantwell, D. (1987). A prospective psychiatric follow-up of children with speech/language disorders. *Journal of the American Academy of Child and Adolescent Psychiatry, 26,* 546–553.

Barnett, W., & Escobar, C. (1990). Economic costs and benefits of early intervention. In S. J. Meisels & J.P. Shonkoff (Eds.), *Handbook of early childhood intervention* (pp. 560–582). New York: Cambridge University Press.

Bates, E. (1976). *Language and context: The acquisition of pragmatics.* San Diego: Academic Press.

Bates, E., O'Connell, B., & Shore, C. (1987). Language and communication in infancy. In J. Osofsky (Ed.), *Handbook of infant development* (pp. 149–203). New York: John Wiley & Sons.

Bloom, L. (1993). *The transition from infancy to language.* New York: Cambridge University Press.

Bronfenbrenner, U. (1979). *The ecology of human development: Experiments by nature and design.* Cambridge, MA: Harvard University Press.

Brooks-Gunn, J., & Duncan, D. (1997). The effects of poverty on children. *The Future of Children, 7*(2), 55–71.

Carnegie Task Force on Meeting the Needs of Young Children. (1994). *Starting Points: Meeting the needs of our youngest children.* New York: Carnegie Corporation of New York.

Cohen, J. (1988). *Statistical power analysis for the behavioral sciences* (2nd ed.). Mahwah, NJ: Lawrence Erlbaum Associates.

Fenson, L., Dale, P., Reznick, S., Thal, D., Bates, E., Hartung, J., Pethick, S., & Reilly, J. (1993). *MacArthur Communicative Development Inventories: User's guide and technical manual.* Baltimore: Paul H. Brookes Publishing Co.

Florida Starting Points. (1997). *Maximizing Florida's brain power: We need to use it or lose it. A collaborative project sponsored by the Carnegie Corporation and the United Way of Florida Success by Six.*

Glascoe, F.P. (1999). The value of parents' concerns to detect and address developmental and behavioural problems. *Journal of Paediatric Child Health, 35,* 1–8.

Harrison, M., & Roush, J. (1996). Age of suspicion, identification and intervention for infants and young children with hearing loss: A national study. *Ear and Hearing, 17,* 55–62.

Hart, B., & Risley, T. (1992). American parenting of language-learning children: Persisting differences in family-child interactions observed in natural home environments. *Developmental Psychology, 28,* 1096–1105.

Howlin, P., & Rutter, M. (1987). The consequences of language delay for other aspects of development. In W. Yule & M. Rutter (Eds.), *Language development and language disorders.* Philadelphia, PA: Lippincott.

Some entries in this bibliography has been reprinted with permission from the First Words web site http://www.firstwords.fsu.edu.

McCathren, R.B., Warren, S.F., & Yoder, P.J. (1996). Prelinguistic predictors of later language development. In K. Cole, P. Dale, & D. Thal (Eds.), *Assessment of communication/language* (pp. 57–75). Baltimore: Paul H. Brookes Publishing Co.

McCathren, R.B., Yoder, P.J., & Warren, S.F. (2000). Testing predictive validity of the Communication Composite of the Communication and Symbolic Behavior Scales. *Journal of Early Intervention, 23*, 36–46.

Meisels, S.J. & Wasik, B.A. (1990). Who should be served? Identifying children in need of early intervention. In S.J. Meisels & J.P. Shonkoff (Eds.), *Handbook of early childhood intervention* (pp. 605–632). New York: Cambridge University Press.

Messick, S.L. (1989). Validity. In R.L. Linn (Ed.), *Educational measurement* (3rd ed., pp. 13–103). New York: American Council on Education/Macmillan.

Mullen, E. (1995). *The Mullen Scales of Early Learning.* Circle Pines, MN: American Guidance Service.

Olswang, L., Rodriguez, B., & Timler, G. (1998). Recommending intervention for toddlers with specific language learning difficulties: We may not have all the answers, but we know a lot. *American Journal of Speech-Language Pathology, 7*, 23–32.

Ounce of Prevention Fund. (1996). *Starting Smart: How early experiences affect brain development.* Chicago: Author.

Parving, A. (1993). Congenital hearing disability: Epidemiology and identification: A comparison between two health authority districts. *International Journal of Pediatric Otolaryngology, 27*, 29–46.

Paul, R. (1991). Profiles of toddlers with slow expressive language development. *Topics in Language Disorders, 11*, 1–13.

Paul, R., & Jennings, P. (1992). Phonological behavior in toddlers with slow expressive language development. *Journal of Speech and Hearing Research, 35*, 99–107.

Paul, R., Looney, S., & Dahm, P. (1991). Communication and socialization skills at ages 2 and 3 in "late-talking" young children. *Journal of Speech and Hearing Research, 34*, 858–865.

Prizant, B., Audet, L., Burke, G., Hummel, L., Maher, S., & Theadore, G. (1990). Communication disorders and emotional/behavioral disorders in children. *Journal of Speech and Hearing Disorders, 55*, 179–192.

Rescorla, L. (1989). The language development survey: A screening tool for delayed language in toddlers.

Rescorla, L., & Alley, A. (2001). Validation of the Language Development Survey (LDS): A Parent report tool for identifying language delay in toddlers. *Journal of Speech, Language, and Hearing Research, 44*, 434–445.

Rescorla, L., & Goosens, M. (1992). Symbolic play development in toddlers with expressive specific language impairment. *Journal of Speech and Hearing Research, 35*, 1290–1302.

Rescorla, L., & Schwartz, E. (1990). Outcome of specific expressive language delay (SELD). *Applied Psycholinguistics, 11*, 393–408.

Salvia, J., & Ysseldyke, J.E. (1988). *Assessment in special and remedial education* (4th ed.). Boston: Houghton Mifflin.

Squires, J., Potter, L., & Bricker, D. (1999). *The ASQ User's Guide for the Ages & Stages Questionnaires: A Parent-Completed, Child-Monitoring System* (2nd ed.). Baltimore: Paul H. Brookes Publishing Co.

Stern, D. (1985). *The interpersonal world of the infant.* New York: Basic Books.

Tabachnick, B., & Fidell, L. (2001). *Using multivariate statistics.* Needham Heights, MA: Allyn & Bacon.

Thal, D., & Tobias, S. (1992). Communicative gestures in children with delayed onset of oral expressive vocabulary. *Journal of Speech and Hearing Research, 35*, 1281–1289.

Thal, D., Tobias, S., & Morrison, D. (1991). Language and gesture in late talkers: A 1-year follow-up. *Journal of Speech and Hearing Research, 34*, 604–612.

U.S. Department of Education. (2000). *Twenty Second Annual Report to Congress on the Implementation of the Individuals with Disabilities Education Act.* (Prepared by the Division of Innovation and Development, Office of Special Education Programs). Washington, DC: U.S. Department of Education.

Walker, D., Greenwood, C.R., Hart, B., & Carta, J. (1994). Prediction of school outcomes based on early language production and socioeconomic factors. *Child Development, 65*, 6–631.

Wetherby, A., Allen, L., Cleary, J., Kublin, K., & Goldstein, H. (in press). Validity and reliability of the Communication and Symbolic Behavior Scales Developmental Profile with very young children. *Journal of Speech, Language, and Hearing Research*

Wetherby, A., Cain, D., Yonclas, D., & Walker, V. (1988). Analysis of intentional communication of normal children from the prelinguistic to the multi-word stage. *Journal of Speech and Hearing Research, 31*, 24–252.

Wetherby, A., & Prizant, B. (1992). Profiling young children's communicative competence. In S. Warren & J. Reichle (Eds.), *Causes and effects in communication and language intervention* (pp. 217–253). Baltimore: Paul H. Brookes Publishing Co.

Wetherby, A., & Prizant, B. (1993). *Communication and Symbolic Behavior Scales, Normed Edition.* Baltimore: Paul H. Brookes Publishing Co.

Wetherby, A., & Prizant, B. (1996). Toward earlier identification of communication and language problems in infants and young children. In S.J. Meisels & E. Fenichel (Eds.), *New visions for the developmental assessment of infants and young children* (pp. 89–312). Washington, DC: Zero to Three/National Center for Infants, Toddlers, & Families.

Wetherby, A., & Prizant, B. (1998). *Communication and Symbolic Behavior Scales Developmental Profile–Research Edition.* Baltimore: Paul H. Brookes Publishing Co.

Wetherby, A. & Prizant, B. (2002). *Communication and Symbolic Behavior Scales Developmental Profile–First Normed Edition.* Baltimore: Paul H. Brookes Publishing Co.

BLANK FORMS A

CSBS DP Infant-Toddler Checklist: Family Information Form

The following information is needed to contact you for follow-up. This information will remain confidential, meaning that it will not be released to anyone without your written permission.

Child's name: _____   Date filled out: _____

Date of birth: _____   Age: _____   Sex: _____

Parent's name: _____

Address: _____

_____

Home phone: _____   Cell phone: _____

Mom's work phone: _____   Dad's work phone: _____

Describe any complications during pregnancy or your child's birth: _____

_____

_____

_____

Was your child born premature: _____ Yes   _____ No

If yes, how many weeks early? _____

Describe any major or recurring health problems your child has had: _____

_____

_____

_____

_____

Describe any concerns you have about your child's development (use back of sheet if needed):

_____

_____

_____

CSBS DP Infant-Toddler Checklist

Child's name: _____ Date of birth: _____ Date filled out: _____

Was birth premature? _____ If yes, how many weeks premature? _____

Filled out by: _____ Relationship to child: _____

Instructions for caregivers: This Checklist is designed to identify different aspects of development in infants and toddlers. Many behaviors that develop before children talk may indicate whether or not a child will have difficulty learning to talk. This Checklist should be completed by a caregiver when the child is between **6 and 24 months of age** to determine whether a referral for an evaluation is needed. The caregiver may be either a parent or another person who nurtures the child daily. Please check all the choices that best describe your child's behavior. If you are not sure, please choose the closest response based on your experience. **Children at your child's age are not necessarily expected to use all the behaviors listed.**

Emotion and Eye Gaze

1. Do you know when your child is happy and when your child is upset?   ☐ Not Yet   ☐ Sometimes   ☐ Often
2. When your child plays with toys, does he/she look at you to see if you are watching?   ☐ Not Yet   ☐ Sometimes   ☐ Often
3. Does your child smile or laugh while looking at you?   ☐ Not Yet   ☐ Sometimes   ☐ Often
4. When you look at and point to a toy across the room, does your child look at it?   ☐ Not Yet   ☐ Sometimes   ☐ Often

Communication

5. Does your child let you know that he/she needs help or wants an object out of reach?   ☐ Not Yet   ☐ Sometimes   ☐ Often
6. When you are not paying attention to your child, does he/she try to get your attention?   ☐ Not Yet   ☐ Sometimes   ☐ Often
7. Does your child do things just to get you to laugh?   ☐ Not Yet   ☐ Sometimes   ☐ Often
8. Does your child try to get you to notice interesting objects—just to get you to look at the objects, not to get you to do anything with them?   ☐ Not Yet   ☐ Sometimes   ☐ Often

Gestures

9. Does your child pick up objects and give them to you?   ☐ Not Yet   ☐ Sometimes   ☐ Often
10. Does your child show objects to you without giving you the object?   ☐ Not Yet   ☐ Sometimes   ☐ Often
11. Does your child wave to greet people?   ☐ Not Yet   ☐ Sometimes   ☐ Often
12. Does your child point to objects?   ☐ Not Yet   ☐ Sometimes   ☐ Often
13. Does your child nod his/her head to indicate *yes*?   ☐ Not Yet   ☐ Sometimes   ☐ Often

Sounds

14. Does your child use sounds or words to get attention or help?   ☐ Not Yet   ☐ Sometimes   ☐ Often
15. Does your child string sounds together, such as *uh oh, mama, gaga, bye bye, bada*?   ☐ Not Yet   ☐ Sometimes   ☐ Often
16. About how many of the following consonant sounds does your child use: *ma, na, ba, da, ga, wa, la, ya, sa, sha*?   ☐ None   ☐ 1–2   ☐ 3–4   ☐ 5–8   ☐ over 8

Words

17. About how many different words does your child use meaningfully that you recognize (such as *baba* for bottle; *gaggie* for doggie)?   ☐ None   ☐ 1–3   ☐ 4–10   ☐ 11–30   ☐ over 30
18. Does your child put two words together (for example, *more cookie, bye bye Daddy*)?   ☐ Not Yet   ☐ Sometimes   ☐ Often

Understanding

19. When you call your child's name, does he/she respond by looking or turning toward you?   ☐ Not Yet   ☐ Sometimes   ☐ Often
20. About how many different words or phrases does your child understand without gestures? For example, if you say "where's your tummy," "where's Daddy," "give me the ball," or "come here," without showing or pointing, your child will respond appropriately.   ☐ None   ☐ 1–3   ☐ 4–10   ☐ 11–30   ☐ over 30

Object Use

21. Does your child show interest in playing with a variety of objects?   ☐ Not Yet   ☐ Sometimes   ☐ Often
22. About how many of the following objects does your child use appropriately: cup, bottle, bowl, spoon, comb or brush, toothbrush, washcloth, ball, toy vehicle, toy telephone?   ☐ None   ☐ 1–2   ☐ 3–4   ☐ 5–8   ☐ over 8
23. About how many blocks (or rings) does your child stack?   **Stacks**   ☐ None   ☐ 2 blocks   ☐ 3–4 blocks   ☐ 5 or more
24. Does your child pretend to play with toys (for example, feed a stuffed animal, put a doll to sleep, put an animal figure in a vehicle)?   ☐ Not Yet   ☐ Sometimes   ☐ Often

Do you have any concerns about your child's development?   ☐ yes   ☐ no   **If yes, please describe on back.**

MANUAL SCORING INSTRUCTIONS FOR THE INFANT-TODDLER CHECKLIST β

The CSBS DP Infant-Toddler Checklist consists of 24 items that range from a total possible of two to four points within each of the seven clusters. The scoring process consists of five steps. The first step is to sum the points for each item to obtain the raw scores for each cluster. The second step is to sum the seven cluster raw scores to obtain the raw scores for each of the three composites. The third step is to add the three composite raw scores to obtain the total raw score. The fourth step is to convert the raw scores to normed scores. The fifth step is to interpret and report the normed scores on the CSBS DP Infant-Toddler Checklist: Screening Report.

Step 1: Sum the points for each item and obtain the raw scores for each of the seven clusters.

Give credit of 0 points for items checked Not Yet, 1 point for items checked Sometimes, or 2 points for items checked Often. For items that describe a series of numbers or ranges, give credit of 0 points for items checked None and 1–4 points for items containing numbered choices. That is, for Items 16 and 22, give credit of 0 points for None, 1 point for 1–2, 2 points for 3–4, 3 points for 5–8, and 4 points for Over 8. For Items 17 and 20, give credit of 0 points for None, 1 point for 1–3, 2 points for 4–10, 3 points for 11–30, and 4 points for Over 30. For Item 23, give credit of 0 points for None, 1 point for 2 blocks, 2 points for 3–4 blocks, and 3 points for 5 or more blocks. The point values and total possible points for each item are listed in Table B.1.

The number of points earned in each cluster should be totaled to yield raw scores. The seven cluster raw scores can be tallied on the CSBS DP Infant-Toddler Checklist to the right of the label for each cluster and then transferred to the left side of the column labeled Raw Score on the CSBS DP Infant-Toddler Checklist: Screening Report. The total possible points for the seven cluster raw scores are listed in Table B.2.

Table B.1.   Point values and total possible points of each item on the Infant-Toddler Checklist

Cluster	Number of items	Possible points	Total possible
Emotion and Eye Gaze Items 1–4	4	2	8
Communication Items 5–8	4	2	8
Gestures Items 9–13	5	2	10
Sounds			
Items 14–15	2	2	4
Item 16	1	4	4
Words			
Item 17	1	4	4
Item 18	1	2	2
Understanding			
Item 19	1	2	2
Item 20	1	4	4
Object Use			
Item 21	1	2	2
Item 22	1	4	4
Item 23	1	3	3
Item 24	1	2	2

Step 2: Sum the seven cluster raw scores to obtain the raw scores for each of the three composites.

The seven clusters are organized into three composites—Social, Speech, and Symbolic. The second step is to sum the seven cluster raw scores to obtain the three composite raw scores. On the CSBS DP Infant-Toddler Checklist: Screening Report, the seven cluster raw scores should be summed to yield the raw scores for the three composites. That is, the raw score for the Social composite is the sum of the Emotion and Eye Gaze, Communication, and Gestures clusters. The raw score for the Speech Composite is the sum of the Sounds and Words clusters. The raw score for the Symbolic Composite is the sum of the Understanding and Object Use clusters. The composite raw scores should be tallied on the right side of the column labeled Raw Score on the Infant-Toddler Checklist: Screening Report. The total possible points for the three composite raw scores are listed in Table B.2.

Step 3: Sum the three composite raw scores to obtain the total raw score.

The third step is to sum the three composite raw scores to obtain the total raw score. On the CSBS DP Infant-Toddler Checklist: Screening Report, the three composite raw scores should be summed to yield the total raw

Table B.2. Total possible points for each cluster, composite, and total on the Infant-Toddler Checklist

Composite	Possible Points
Social Composite	
Emotion and Eye Gaze	8
Communication	8
Gestures	<u>10</u>
Total	**26**
Speech Composite	
Sounds	8
Words	<u>6</u>
Total	**14**
Symbolic Composite	
Understanding	6
Object Use	<u>11</u>
Total	**17**
Social Composite	26
Speech Composite	14
Symbolic Composite	<u>17</u>
Total	**57**

score. The total raw score should be tallied on the right side of the column labeled Raw Score on the Infant-Toddler Checklist: Screening Report, just below the composite raw scores. The total possible points for the total raw score are listed in Table B.2.

Step 4: Convert the composite and total raw scores to normed scores.

The fourth step is to convert the composite and total raw scores to normed scores. Normed scores are provided in the norms tables for the CSBS DP Infant-Toddler Checklist in Appendix C and are based on chronological age to reflect the performance of children in the standardization sample by 1-month intervals from 6 to 24 months. Use the following steps to compute the child's chronological age:

1. Enter the child's name, date filled out, and date of birth on the CSBS DP Infant-Toddler Checklist: Screening Report. If the child is more than 4 weeks premature, make sure to enter the child's corrected date of birth and indicate this by writing corrected in parentheses after the date of birth and chronological age.

2. Compute the child's chronological age on the CSBS DP Infant-Toddler Checklist: Screening Report by subtracting the child's date of birth or if the child is more than 4 weeks premature, corrected date of birth (month, day, and year) from the date of completion (month, day, and year).

3. Subtract days first, then months, then years. Table B.3 shows a simple subtraction in which no borrowing is required.

4. If the day of the month on which the child was born is larger than the day of the month of testing, borrow 30 days; that is, add 30 days to the day of testing and subtract 1 month from the month of testing. If necessary, also borrow 1 month of testing by adding 12 months to the actual month of testing and subtracting 1 year from the testing year. Table B.4 shows a subtraction in which borrowing is required to calculate chronological age for a child whose date of completion was November 5, 2000.

5. The child's chronological age should be reported in months, and the month should not be rounded up. For example, a child is 12 months old from 12 months and 0 days until that child turns 13 months and 0 days. To calculate age in months, first multiply the number of years by 12, and then add the number of extra months. The chronological age for the child in Table B.3 is 16 months (i.e., multiply 1 for the number of years by 12, and add 4 extra months to get 16) and would not be rounded to 17 months, even though the child is more than 16½ months old. The chronological age for the child in Table B.4 is 9 months. Standard scores and percentile ranks are the normed scores provided in the norms tables for the composites and total of the CSBS DP Infant-Toddler Checklist in Appendix C. The standard scores for the three composites are based on a mean of 10 and a standard deviation of 3. The standard scores for the total are based on a mean of 100 and a standard deviation of 15. Because standard scores reflect equal units of measurement, they may be added, subtracted, or averaged. A percentile rank reflects the percentage of children in the sample scoring at or below a given raw score. Percentile ranks, unlike standard scores, should not be added, subtracted, or averaged. Standard scores, rather than percentile ranks, should be used to reflect average performance, whether it is the average of several scores for an individual child or the average of scores obtained from a group of children. The relationship between the standard scores for the composites and total and percentile ranks is shown in Table B.5.

Once the child's chronological age is known, use the following steps to look up the standard scores and percentile ranks for the composite and total raw scores.

1. Use the norms tables for the CSBS DP Infant-Toddler Checklist in Appendix C. On the table for the Social Composite, find the column

Table B.3. Calculating chronological age without needing to borrow

	Month	Day	Year
Date of completion	10	25	2000
Date of birth	6	4	1999
Chronological age	**4**	**21**	**1**
CSBS DP age	**16**		

Table B.4. Calculating chronological age with borrowing

	Month	Day	Year
Date of completion	~~11~~10	~~5~~35	2000
Date of birth	1	28	2000
Chronological age	**9**	**7**	**0**
CSBS DP age	**9**		

Table B.5.   Standard deviations (SD), standard scores (SS), and percentile ranks (%ile) for the composites and total scores

SD	Composite SS	Total SS	%ile
	17	135	99
+2 SD	16	130	98
	15	125	95
	14	120	91
+1 SD	13	115	84
	12	110	75
	11	105	63
Mean	10	100	50
	9	95	37
	8	90	25
−1 SD	7	85	16
	6	80	9
	5	75	5
−2 SD	4	70	2
	3	65	1

with the child's chronological age in months, read down the column until you find the child's Social Composite raw score, and look to the left to find the corresponding standard score (SS) and percentile (%ile) rank. Enter these scores in the appropriate columns on the CSBS DP Infant-Toddler Checklist: Screening Report.

2.   Repeat this for the Speech Composite, the Symbolic Composite, and the total raw scores.

Step 5: Interpret and report the normed scores on the CSBS DP Infant-Toddler Checklist: Screening Report.

The fifth and last step is to interpret and report the normed scores on the CSBS DP Infant-Toddler Checklist: Screening Report. Once the child's standard scores and percentile ranks are entered, use the following steps to determine if the normed scores are of concern and to decide what to recommend.

1.   Determine if the normed scores are of concern and enter Yes in the column labeled "Concern." Leave blank if the child is at or above criterion level. Four scores may fall in a range of concern or no concern—the three composite scores and the total score. We have set the criterion level for concern for the composite and total scores based on performance of at least 1.25 standard deviations below the mean as follows:

• Standard scores at or below 6 for the composite scores

• Standard scores at or below 81 for the total score

• Percentile ranks at or below the 10th for the composites and total scores

2. Make a recommendation on the bottom of the CSBS DP Infant-Toddler Checklist: Screening Report by checking one of the three boxes. Based on our validation studies summarized in Chapter 3, we have determined that the following recommendation should be made, depending on the child's pattern of scores:

- A child should be referred for an evaluation if the Social Composite, Symbolic Composite, or the Total Score are in the concern range.

- A child should be monitored carefully if the Speech Composite is in the concern range and should be referred for an evaluation if in the concern range on a second Checklist completed 3 months later.

It is recommended that the Checklist be used to monitor development every 3 months between 6 and 24 months of age. Because it is based on parent report, it is possible for the caregiver to overestimate or underestimate the child's abilities. Therefore, this tool should be used along with a brief observation of the child by a health care or child care service provider. Children who have scores in the concern range on any composite or on the total score may have specific language impairments, hearing impairments, more general developmental delays, or autism spectrum disorder. With further development, these children may only have speech impairments or they may catch up to children their age. The Checklist should only be used to decide that a developmental evaluation is needed. Caution should be taken not to alarm parents. We find that many parents already have concerns about their child, especially as their child is approaching age 18 months and is behind in language development. The early intervention literature emphasizes the notion of multiple risk factors; therefore, a child's scores on this Checklist need to be considered in relation to other known biological or environmental risk factors.

Clinical judgment should be used in making decisions about the need for further evaluation with these cutoffs as guidelines. Remember that the Checklist is not meant for a diagnostic evaluation and should not be used for a differential diagnosis.

NORMS TABLES FOR THE CSBS DP INFANT-TODDLER CHECKLIST

C

INFANT-TODDLER CHECKLIST SOCIAL COMPOSITE SCORES

SS	%ile	6	7	8	9	10	11	12	13	14	15	16	17	18	19	20	21	22	23	24
n =		50	42	77	126	86	312	296	121	128	174	98	99	133	107	84	87	82	50	36
	Age (months)	6	7	8	9	10	11	12	13	14	15	16	17	18	19	20	21	22	23	24
17	99	17-26	20-26	22-26	25-26	26	26	26	26	26	26	26	26	26	26	26	26	26	26	26
16	98		18-19	21	22-24	23-25	25	25	25	25	25	25	25							
15	95	15-16	15-17	19-20	20-21	22	24	24	24	24										
14	91	14	14	18	19	20-21	23	23	23											
13	84	13		17	17-18	19														
12	75	11-12	13	15-16	16	18	21-22	22	22	23	24	24	24	25	25	25	25	25	25	25
11	63	10	12	13-14	14-15	17	20	20-21	21	22	23	23	23	24	24	24	24	24	24	24
10	50		11	12	13	16	18-19	19	20	21	22	22	22	22-23	23	23	23	23	23	23
9	37	9	10	11	12	15	17	18	19	20	20-21	21	21	21	21-22	22	22	22	22	22
8	25	8	9	9-10	10-11	14	15-16	16-17	17-18	18-19	19	19-20	20	20	20	20-21	20-21	20-21	21	21
7	16		8	8	9	12-13	13-14	14-15	15-16	16-17	18	18	18-19	18-19	18-19	19	19	19	20	20
6	9	7	7	7	8	10-11	10-12	12-13	13-14	15	16-17	16-17	16-17	17	17	17-18	18	18	19	19
5	5	6	6	6	7	8-9	8-9	10-11	11-12	14	14-15	15	15	16	16	16	17	17	17-18	18
4	2	5	5		6	6-7	7	8-9	9-10	9-13	11-13	11-14	13-14	14-15	15	15	15-16	16	16	17
3	1	0-4	0-4	0-5	0-5	0-5	0-6	0-7	0-8	0-8	0-10	0-10	0-12	0-13	0-14	0-14	0-14	0-15	0-15	0-16

SEM 1.1

68% Confidence Interval ± 1.1

90% Confidence Interval ± 1.8

95% Confidence Interval ± 2.1

INFANT-TODDLER CHECKLIST SPEECH COMPOSITE SCORES

SS	%ile	6	7	8	9	10	11	12	13	14	15	16	17	18	19	20	21	22	23	24
n =	Age (months)	50	42	77	126	86	312	296	121	128	174	98	99	133	107	84	87	82	50	36
17	99	8-14	8-14	10-14	11-14	12-14	13-14	13-14	13-14	13-14	14	14	14	14	14	14	14	14	14	14
16	98	7	7	9	10	11	12	12	12	12	13	13	13	13	13	13	13		13	
15	95	6	6	8	9	10	11	11	11	11	12	12			12					
14	91			7	8	9	10	10	10		11									
13	84				7															
12	75	5	5	6	6	8	9	9	9	10	10	11	12	12	13	13	13	13	13	13
11	63	4	4	5	5	7	8	8	8	9	9	10	11	11	12	12	12	12	12	12
10	50	3	3	4	4	6	7	7	7	8	8	9	10	10	10-11	11	11	11	10-11	11
9	37	2					6			7		8	9	9	9	10	10	10		
8	25											8								
7	16	1	2	3	3	5	5	6	6	6	7	7	7-8	8	8	8-9	9	9	9	10
6	9	0	1	2	2	4	4	5	5	5	6	6	6	6-7	7	7	7-8	7-8	8	9
5	5		0	1		2-3	3	4	4	4	5	5	5	5	6	6	6	6	7	8
4	2			0		0-1		3	3			4	4	4	4-5	5	5		6	7
3	1				0-1	0-1	0-2	0-2	0-2	0-3	0-3	0-3	0-3	0-3	0-3	0-4	0-4	0-5	0-5	0-6

SEM 1.0

68% Confidence Interval ±1.0   90% Confidence Interval ±1.7   95% Confidence Interval ±2.0

INFANT-TODDLER CHECKLIST SYMBOLIC COMPOSITE SCORES

SS	%ile	6	7	8	9	10	11	12	13	14	15	16	17	18	19	20	21	22	23	24
n =		50	42	77	126	86	312	296	121	128	174	98	99	133	107	84	87	82	50	36
17	99	9-17	9-17	11-17	11-17	14-17	15-17	16-17	16-17	16-17	16-17	17	17	17	17	17	17	17	17	17
16	98	7-8	8	10	10	12-13	14	15	15	15		16	16	16	16	16				
15	95	6	7	9	9	11	13	14	14		15				16	16	16	16	16	16
14	91			8		10		13		14	14	15	15					15	15	
13	84			7		9		12	10	11	13	14	14	15	15	15	15	15	14	16
12	75	5	6	6	7	8	11	11	12	13	13		13	14	14	14	14	12-13	13	14
11	63		5	5			10		11	12	12	14	14	14	14		11	11	12	
10	50	4	4		6	7	9	10	10	11	13	13	13	14	13	11	10	10	11	13
9	37						8	9		11	13					9-10	10			12
8	25	3	3	4	5	6	7	8	9	10	10	12	12	12	13	11	11	9	14	14
7	16											11	11	11	11-12	12	12	12-13	13	13
6	9	2	2	3		5	6	7	8	9	9	9-10	10	10-9	9	9-10	10	11	12	12
5	5	1		2		4	5	6	7	6	6-8	7-8	8-9	8-9	8	9-10	10	10	11	11
4	2	0	2	2	3	3	4	5	6	6	5	6	7	7	8	8	8-9	9	9-10	11
3	1		0-1	0-1	0-2	0-2	0-3	0-3	0-4	0-4	0-4	0-5	0-6	0-6	0-7	0-7	0-7	0-8	0-8	0-10

SEM 1.1

68% Confidence Interval ± 1.1

90% Confidence Interval ± 1.8

95% Confidence Interval ± 2.1

INFANT-TODDLER CHECKLIST TOTAL SCORES

SS	%ile	6	7	8	9	10	11	12	13	14	15	16	17	18	19	20	21	22	23	24
n =	Age (months)	50	42	77	126	86	312	296	121	128	174	98	99	133	107	84	87	82	50	36
135	99	33-57	34-57	38-57	45-57	50-57	52-57	52-57	53-57	54-57	55-57	56-57	56-57	57	57	57	57	57	57	57
134	99					48-49	51				54	55	55	56						
133	99					48-49	50													
132	98														56					
131	98	32				47		51												
130	98		33		44	42-46	49	50	52	53	53					56				
129	97		32	37	40-43			49	51	52										
128	97				39		48		50					55						
127	96	26-30			37-38		47		50								56			
126	96		30-31	36	36	40		48	49											
125	95		29	35							52									
124	95	24	28	34	35	39	46	47	48				54		55	55			56	
123	94	23	27	33	34	38	45	46	47									56		
122	93																			
121	92																			
120	91	22	26	32				45	46	50	51		53	54	54		55	55	55	56
119	90		25	31	33		44			50										
118	89															54				
117	87					37		44					52	53	53					
116	86				32		43			49	49	51								
115	84																			55
114	83	21	24	30	31	36	42	43	45	48	48						54	54	54	
113	81				30	35				47										
112	79			29	29		41	42			47		51				53			
111	77													52	52					
110	75					34	40	41	43	46	46	50						53		54
109	73					33	39	40												
108	70	20	23	28	28		38		42	45		49	50		50		52	52	53	
107	68		22	27																53
106	66													51					52	
105	63		21	26	27		37	39	41	44	44	48	49	51		51				
104	61		20	25	26			38					48	51			51	51	51	
103	58	19		24	25	31	36		40	43	43	48		50	49	50	50	50	53	53
102	55	18		23						42				49						52
101	53	17										47	47	48		49				51
100	50				24		35	37	39	41		46		47			50	50	50	50

(continued)

INFANT-TODDLER CHECKLIST TOTAL SCORES *(continued)*

SS	%ile	n=50	42	77	126	86	312	296	121	128	174	98	99	133	107	84	87	82	50	36
	Age (months)	6	7	8	9	10	11	12	13	14	15	16	17	18	19	20	21	22	23	24
99	47	16		22												48				50
98	45		19		23							45	46		48		49			49
97	42						34	36	38	40	42			46	47	47		49		48
96	40				22														49	
95	37					30	33	35				44	45	45	46	46	48			47
94	35	15	18				32	34	36	39	41			44	45	45	47	48	48	
93	32		17	21	21															
92	30			20								43	44	43	44	44	46	47	47	
91	27																			
90	25			19	20	29	31	33	35	38	40	42	42-43	42	43	43	45	46	46	
89	23	14	16			28	30	32	34	37	39	41	41	41	42	42	44	45	45	46
88	21		15		20		29	31	33	36	38	40	40	40	41	41	43	44	44	45
87	19			18					32											44
86	18				19															
85	16			17		27	28	30	31	35	37	39	39	39	40	40	42	43	43	
84	14	13	14				27	29	30	34	36	38	38	38	39	39	41	42	42	43
83	13			16		26	26	28	29		35	37	37	37	38	38	40	41	41	42
82	12				18		25	27	28	33	34	36	36	36	37	37	39	40	40	41
81	10				17	25														
80	9		13				24	24-26	26-27	32	33	35	35	35	35-36	36	38	39	39	
79	8			15		24	23	23	25	31	32	34	33-34	34	34	35	37	38	38	40
78	7			14		23	22	22	24	30	31	33	32	33	33	34	36	37		39
77	6					22	21	21	23	29	30	32	31	32	32	33	35	36	36-37	
76	6																			
75	5	12		13		20-21	20	20	22		29	31	30	31	31	32	34	35		
74	4	11	12		15	19			21	23-28	28	30	29	30	29-30	31	33			38
73	4	10	11	12		18			20	22	27		28		28	30	32	33-34	35	37
72	3	9		11	13-14	17	18-19	18-19	19	20-21	23-26	28-29	27	28-29	27	29	31	32		36
71	3				12		17	17				27	26	27						
70	2		10	10		16	16	16	18	19	21	23-26	25	26	26	28	30	31	33-34	
69	2	8																		35
68	2																			
67	1		9		10-11	11-15	13-15		17	17-18	20					27	29			
66	1		8	9	9		13-15					22								
65	1																			
SEM 4.0		0-7	0-7	0-8	0-8	0-10	0-12	0-15	0-16	0-16	0-19	0-21	0-24	0-25	0-25	0-26	0-28	0-30	0-32	0-34

68% Confidence Interval ± 4.0

90% Confidence Interval ± 6.6

95% Confidence Interval ± 7.8

FREQUENTLY ASKED QUESTIONS (FAQs) ABOUT THE EASY-SCORE PROGRAM

What do I need to run the Easy-Score program?

To use the Easy-Score program on a Microsoft Windows platform, users need the following minimum equipment and software:

an Intel compatible 486/33 PC or higher
at least 16 MB of RAM
a hard disk with at least 20 MB of free space
a CD-ROM drive
Windows 95 or later, with Internet Explorer 4.0 or later, or
   Windows NT 4.0 (with Service Pack 3 or later)

Note: The application requires the shfolder.dll and comctl32.dll files, which are installed by Windows NT 4.0 with Service Pack 3 (or later) or by Internet Explorer 4.0 (or later).

Note: The Easy-Score program is not available for use on Macintosh computers.

How do I install Easy-Score?

Place the CD-ROM into the disk drive. Wait. The CD will start automatically. Follow the steps on screen. Please refer to the Software License and Support Agreement in Appendix E of the User's Manual. If the setup does not automatically initiate, then at your desktop, double click on the My Computer icon. Next, double click on the icon for your CD-ROM drive (this can be any letter from D though Z). Then double-click on setup.exe and the program will begin the installation process.

I don't have enough hard disk space to install.

Review the system requirements above. Exit installation and free up more disk space. For example, empty your recycle bin. If you use compression software, check your real disk space.

My system freezes during installation.

Close any open applications, restart your computer, and try installing Easy-Score. Review the memory requirements above. For help with troubleshooting your PC's memory, choose Help from the Windows Start menu and enter "memory, troubleshooting."

How do I move data from one computer to another?

The best method for moving Easy-Score data from one computer to another is to back up the complete directory that was created during the installation process. Unless you chose to install Easy-Score somewhere other than the default, the path should be C:\Program Files\CSBS DP Infant-Toddler Checklist and Easy-Score. You should find 28 different files in this folder. Either use a backup utility to back the directory up to tape or use a Read/Write CD-ROM drive and copy the directory to a blank CD.

How do I back up and then restore my Easy-Score file? My database records?

Either use a backup utility to back the directory up to tape or use a Read/Write CD-ROM drive and copy the directory to a blank CD. Unless you chose to install Easy-Score somewhere other than the default, the path should be C:\Program Files\CSBS DP Infant-Toddler Checklist and Easy-Score. You should find 28 different files in this folder. These files may be backed up and restored wherever you need them.

How do I delete existing database records?

Because deleting records is a very permanent thing in Easy-Score, you may only delete one record at a time. You may do this from the screen where you view an existing Easy-Score record. To delete, do a search and find the record you want to delete. On the first review screen, which looks very much like the initial Child Information Screen, there is a delete button.

How do I get answers to my technical questions?

Technical questions may be addressed to support@TECHeGROUP.com or by calling (800) 830-3387 9:00 A.M. to 5:00 P.M. EST. Your call will be returned as soon as possible.

SOFTWARE LICENSE AND SUPPORT AGREEMENT

Please read this Software License and Services Agreement ("Agreement") carefully before installing or using the software. This Agreement gives you, the customer, certain benefits, rights, and obligations. By installing or using the software, you are accepting the terms and conditions of this Agreement between you and Paul H. Brookes Publishing Co., Inc. ("Brookes Publishing Co."). If you do not agree to the terms and conditions in this Agreement, return the User's Guide, unopened disc, and any accompanying print materials within thirty (30) days to Brookes Publishing Co. with a copy of the invoice or packing slip from Brookes Publishing Co. for a full refund of the purchase price. If you purchased this software from a source other than Brookes Publishing Co., please contact that reseller for information on your returns privileges.

Definitions

For purposes of this Agreement, "Software" is defined as the Brookes computer program with which this Agreement is included and any updates or maintenance releases thereto. To "use" the Software means storing, loading, installing, executing, and displaying the Software. The terms "you," "your," "user," or "customer" are synonymous and refer to someone who purchases a license for the Software from Brookes Publishing Co. or from a Brookes-authorized reseller. Someone so purchasing the Software is an "authorized user." A "software support number" is provided to you at the time you purchase the Software and is a non-transferable identification number that gives you access to assistance in the use of this Software as described in the "Services and Support" section of this Agreement.

License

1. Brookes Publishing Co. licenses and authorizes you to use the Software on a microcomputer located within your facilities. This license is granted on a limited, non-exclusive, non-transferable basis for use of the Software on a single computer. If the Software is licensed for "concurrent use" or "site use," you may not allow more than the maximum number of authorized users to use the Software concurrently. To inquire

about a "concurrent use" license, contact the Brookes Publishing Subsidiary Rights Department at perms@brookespublishing.com or at either of the telephone numbers listed below in the "Services and Support" section of this Agreement.

2. You agree that you will abide by the Copyright Law of the United States of America. Copyright, trademark, and other laws protect the Software in its entirety. The law provides you with the right to make one back-up copy. It prohibits you from making more than one copy, except as expressly allowed by Brookes Publishing Co. In the event that the Software is protected against copying in such a way that it cannot be duplicated, Brookes Publishing Co. will provide you with one back-up copy at minimal cost or no charge. You agree that you will not give, rent, lend, resell, or distribute a copy of the Software to any other person; duplicate the Software by any other means, including electronic transmission; make the Software available for any file-sharing service; electronically send the Software to any other person; or copy the print materials or user documentation accompanying the Software. If you received the Software through any of the means specified here, you are not authorized to use the Software.

3. You also agree that you will not prepare derivative works based on the Software. Such action is not permitted under Copyright Law. For example, you cannot prepare an alternative hardware version or format based on the Software. If you believe you are entitled to make an alternative format of the Software because you have a disability and require access by other means, please contact the Brookes Publishing Subsidiary Rights Department at perms@brookespublishing.com for written authorization.

4. You acknowledge that the Software is subject to regulation by agencies of the United States government, including the U.S. Department of Commerce, which prohibits export or diversion of certain technical products to certain countries. You will comply in all respects with all export and re-export restrictions applicable to the Software, its documentation, and related materials.

Ownership

The Software is owned, copyrighted, and trademarked by Brookes Publishing Co. Your license confers no title or ownership in the Software and is not a sale or grant of any rights in the Software. Brookes Publishing Co. may protect its rights in the event of any violation of this Agreement.

Services and Support

Brookes Publishing Co. uses a variety of methods (e.g., in-product, Internet, fax, and telephone) to provide customers with product-specific and technical support to in connection with the Software.

The User's Guide for this Software provides step-by-step instructions so that you can quickly and easily find the information you need. If you have questions about the product, you can often find an answer by using this manual.

Product-Specific Support

If the User's Guide is unable to answer your questions about the *CSBS DP Infant-Toddler Checklist*, or if you would like to purchase additional copies of the User's Guide, contact:

Brookes Publishing Co.
P.O.Box 10624
Baltimore, MD 21285-0624
Phone: 800-638-3775 (from the U.S.A. or Canada) or 410-337-9580 (worldwide) (8:00 a.m to 5:00 pm. Eastern Time)
E-mail: custserv@brookespublishing.com
Web: www.brookespublishing.com/csbsdp

Technical Support

If the User's Guide is unable to answer your questions about the installation or operation of the *Easy-Score* program, then for technical support that is software related, contact:

TechE-Group
535 Madison Avenue, Suite 404
Covington, KY 41011
U.S.A.
Phone: 800-830-3387 (9:00 a.m. to 5:00 p.m. Central Time)
E-mail: destewart@TechEGroup.com
Web: www.TechEGroup.com

Users contacting TechE-Group must provide their "software support number" to receive assistance. Your software support number is an identification number unique to each authorized user that is packed with the Software at the time of purchase. With the software support number, authorized users are entitled to a certain level of complimentary support for technical questions. TechE-Group may also provide additional user assistance for a fee. Users should refer to the Brookes Publishing web site www.brookespublishing.co/csbsdp or contact TechE-Group through any of the means listed above for the details of this additional user assistance. The terms and conditions governing the offering of both product-specific and technical support related to this Software, some of which may have fees chargeable to you, are announced by Brookes Publishing Co. from time to time. Consult www.brookespublishing.co/csbsdp for the most current information on services and support available to authorized users, as well as for information on any updates to the Software.

Limited Warranty

If you have a problem with the operation of the Software or believe the disc on which the Software is stored is defective, please contact Brookes Publishing Co. about securing a replacement. We cannot, however, offer free replacements of discs damaged through normal wear and tear, or lost while in your possession. Nor does Brookes Publishing Co. warrant that the Software will satisfy your requirements, that the operation of the Software will be uninterrupted or error-free, or that program defects in the Software can be corrected. Except as described in this Agreement, Software and discs are distributed "as is" without warranties of any kind either express or implied, including but not limited to implied warranties of merchantability and fitness for a particular purpose or use. Some states do not allow limitations on the duration of an implied warranty so the above limitation or exclusion might not apply to you. This warranty gives you specific legal rights, and you might have other rights that vary from state to state, or province to province.

The remedies in this warranty are your sole and exclusive remedies. Except as indicated above, in no event will Brookes Publishing Co. be liable for loss of data or for direct, special, incidental, consequential, or other damage, whether based on breach of contract, breach of warranty, tort, product liability, or otherwise. Some states or provinces do not allow the exclusion or limitation of incidental or consequential damages, so the above limitation or exclusion may not apply to you.

The limitations of damages or liability set forth in this Agreement are fundamental elements of the bargain between Brooks Publishing Co. and you. You acknowledge and agree that Brookes Publishing Co. would not be able to provide this product on an economic basis without such limitations.

Termination

Brookes Publishing Co. may automatically terminate your license to use this Software for failure to comply with any of the terms of this Agreement. Upon termination, you must immediately destroy the Software, User's Guide, and any other accompanying print materials.

Miscellaneous

This Agreement does not limit any rights that Brookes Publishing Co. may have under trade secret, copyright, trademark, patent, or other laws. The agents, employees, and distributors of Brookes Publishing Co. are not authorized to make modifications to this Agreement, or to make any additional representations, commitments, or warranties binding on Brookes Publishing Co. If any provision of this Agreement is invalid or unenforceable under applicable law, then it shall be, to that extent, deemed omitted and the remaining provisions will continue in full force and effect. The validity and performance of this Agreement shall be governed by Maryland law and applicable federal law.

INDEX

Page numbers followed by *f* indicate figures; those followed by *t* indicate tables.

Communication and Symbolic Behavior Scales Developmental Profile (CSBS DP)™ Order Form

ORDER THE COMPLETE CSBS DP™ SYSTEM AND SAVE $60!

Includes Test Kit & Toy Kit

Quantity

____ **Complete CSBS DP™, First Normed Edition**
Manual, Toy Kit, Forms Package, Sampling Video (VHS), Scoring Video (VHS), and carrying bag
Stock #5494 / Price: $399.00

Quantity

____ **CSBS DP™ Test Kit, First Normed Edition**—Manual, 25 Infant-Toddler Checklists, 25 Infant-Toddler Checklist: Screening Reports, 25 Caregiver Questionnaires, 25 Caregiver Questionnaire: Scoring Worksheets, 25 Caregiver Perceptions Ratings, 25 Behavior Sample Worksheets, 1 Outline of Sampling Procedures and Instructions card, 1 Sampling Video, 1 Scoring Video / Stock #5516 / Price: $199.95

____ **CSBS DP™ Toy Kit**—(For owners of CSBS™: All the toys needed to implement CSBS DP™ are included in the CSBS™ Toy Kit) / Stock #5524 / Price: $259.95

TEST KIT ELEMENTS ALSO SOLD SEPERATELY

____ **CSBS DP™ Manual, First Normed Edition**
Stock #5567 / Price: $65.00

____ **CSBS DP™ Forms, First Normed Edition**—25 Infant-Toddler Checklists, 25 Infant-Toddler Checklist: Screening Reports, 25 Caregiver Questionnaires, 25 Caregiver Questionnaire: Scoring Worksheets, 25 Caregiver Perceptions Ratings, 25 Behavior Sample Worksheets, and 1 Outline of Sampling Procedures and Instructions card
Stock #5540 / Price: $35.00

____ **CSBS DP™ Caregiver Questionnaire**—Package of 50 with 50 scoring worksheets / Stock #6369 / Price: $25.00

____ **CSBS DP™ Sampling Video**—Stock #5575 / Price: $50.00

____ **CSBS DP™ Scoring Video**—Stock #5583 / Price: $50.00

CSBS DP™ Infant-Toddler Checklist and Easy-Score CD-ROM

This scoring software includes a complete copy of the **Checklist** and comes with a **User's Guide**. User input responses from the completed **Checklist** and the program calculates composite percentiles and standard scores based on embedded norms. It also generates a screening report for clinicians to add to the child's health record, and the clinician can select from a menu of three letters to share personalized results and recommendations with the family.

____ **CSBS DP™ Infant-Toddler Checklist and Easy-Score**—PC-compatible CD-ROM, with User's Guide
Stock #5605 / Price: $99.95

To order call toll-free **1-800-638-3775** (8 A.M.–5 P.M., ET U.S. and CAN)
or **410-337-9580** (worldwide); or order online at
www.brookespublishing.com